James Jones, MD, PhD, MHA credentials are exceptional for understanding and giving the reader a heads up for a healthy life. He was an honor society student in medical school and when earning a PhD in Cell Biology. He was a professor teaching and doing research in several medical schools.

He has written 400 medical articles and four books. Being retired, he wrote health matters articles for two local magazines. Now after four decades of gaining understanding of the usual misconceptions ordinary people make about their body and health, he wishes to offer wholesome counsel to help reengineer a gratifying way of life.

James Jones, MD, PhD, MHA

HEALTHIER LIVING

AUSTIN MACAULEY PUBLISHERS™

LONDON • CAMBRIDGE • NEW YORK • SHARJAH

Ordering Information
Quantity sales: Special discounts are available on quantity purchases by corporations, associations, and others. For details, contact the publisher at the address below.

Publisher's Cataloging-in-Publication data
Jones, MD, PhD, MHA, James
Healthier Living

ISBN 9798891551374 (Paperback)
ISBN 9798891551381 (Hardback)
ISBN 9798891551398 (ePub e-book)

Library of Congress Control Number: 2023923749

www.austinmacauley.com/us

First Published 2024
Austin Macauley Publishers LLC
40 Wall Street, 33rd Floor, Suite 3302
New York, NY 10005
USA

mail-usa@austinmacauley.com
+1 (646) 5125767

Table of Contents

The Healthy Concept of Health

What is most important subject matter in a person's material life? Frequently, family, finances, occupation, and other aspects of life are mentioned. Health seems rarely considered, but if one or a loved one becomes ill, that illness edges into first place and everything else lags behind. The focus of life is to be successful morally, academically, financially, and with relationships.

The overwhelming focus of health is on not becoming sick. Most responses to questions about staying healthy are simply eat right and exercise.

Why do we not understand the essentials of health better? We neglect health because we too often loosely grasp the most important things in our life as knee-jerk responses, without thinking; they just happen. Health is the water in our swimming pool; being the one most important thing, without which, it would not be a swimming pool.

We pay attention to the solid material of our "pool" (our body), not the life it contains—overlooking the essential thing. We ignore its importance because, as the water in our swimming pool, it is just there. Many pool owners hire people knowledgeable in pool water's care; they only have vague and non-specific knowledge about pool water.

In our lives, we get pool water people when the water is defiled, when the ideal is to keep it from becoming fouled. However, each of us must maintain our life processes and must know specifically how to do so.

The word "health" derives from Old English roots meaning wholeness or the state of being uninjured. Originally, the word meant, "being fit" for life—having health was a good omen for all of one's activities. Wellbeing is a near synonym. Health's meaning, however, currently has abridged to mean freedom from physical maladies. To accept that flawed conviction is to fail to aspire to having really good everyday lives. Oh no!

The World Health Organization defines health as 'A state of complete physical, mental, and social wellbeing and not merely the absence of disease or infirmity.' Health worsens with illness, yet, is incompletely defined by absence of disease that defines minimalist or subsistence health. Instead, the Army's slogan, "be the best you can be" notion applies to each individual's state of health. Pay attention!

Above all else, health is a gauge of functionality; it is loosely termed "fitness". Be fit! Health increases or decreases as a person's ability to function changes. That is the healthy concept of health. Athletes and soldiers undergo rigorous physical training to improve physical fitness. I was never as physically healthy as when in the military.

Rosy cheeks, muscular build, pleasant countenance, and energetic behaviors are superficial evidence of physical health. In reality, their importance is signaling strength and endurance functionality. They are acquired by health promoting activities.

Healthiness is attained or lost incrementally, usually in small unappreciated bits. Incremental changes that accumulate are very powerful over time. The Grand Canyon was sculpted over time—by handfuls. Amazing indeed! Professors gained knowledge a page at a time and athletes don't just show up for games. Every happening results from a cause which is a saying we apply everywhere except our health.

Health is qualitative and divisible into different aspects. Because the majority of threats to health are physical or mental in nature, those aspects are considered the primary determinants of health. Emotional, social, occupational, financial, and spiritual health aspects are important as well. Each contributes or detracts from the others and determines our emotional status.

Health maintenance has many aspects the necessary knowledge is going to be presented in the following health articles. Some aspects may be found at the author's website, drjimshealthtips.com. Enjoy and get with the program.

Let's Focus Vociferously on Health Literacy

The determinant that positively correlates with an individual's cost of healthcare is health literacy. A number of first-rate medical studies show feeble health literacy is associated with second-rate utilization of health care services, substantially higher costs, and even worse, poorer outcomes. OMG!

After all, we are the instigators of our health care, not the insurers, docs, and certainly not the government. In this available space, I shall focus on the most obvious health literacy cost issues.

The Institute of Medicine is one of the most authoritative sources of medical related info. This is how they define health literacy: 'The degree to which individuals have the capacity to obtain, process, and understand basic health information and services needed to make appropriate health decisions.' AMEN!

The cost of medical care varies considerably and more costly often does not mean superior. Clearly, one does not want to scrimp concerning their health but paying more for the same products or services is not the way to conduct your medical care delivery.

Generic drugs' prices average 20% of brand-named ones because they don't share the cost of development and FDA approval which is multiple millions of dollars. Are generic users settling for less quality? No, not at all! The FDA has stringent criteria for approval of generic medications. In extensive testing, the chemical composition of active ingredients must be identical, and the absorption must be the same.

This means the drug works the same way and is absorbed in the same amount. Over 2,000 generic's absorptions into the body were compared to the costly ones and the generics averaged 96.5%, which provides the same clinical results as the brand name. Further, in dozens of medical studies, outcomes were compared and in every study were identical. **Go generic**.

Comparison shopping is always a levelheaded approach, especially in regard to repetitive needs. Forget the most convenience paramount routine; the closest pharmacy may be more expensive. Even check to see how online pharmacies match up with prices.

Also, compare the prices when buying over-the-counter meds. Usually if the brand is the store's where you are purchasing the meds, the price will be lower.

There are several no-win situations with health insurance: find out if your insurance has a network of physicians and hospitals where you pay more if they are out of network. This is especially true when emergency care is needed. There is little worry when one has medicare coverage; those providing care to seniors essentially have no choice but to accept because of the vast number of enrollees—currently 65.7 million and continuing to rise.

If you need care before you can get an appointment, there are two choices: urgent care or emergency care. Suddent, possibly serious, situations such as chest pain or a serious fall need an emergency room visit. However, relative minor situations such as a sore throat or bad cold can be treated effectively at an urgent care office. The urgent care visit will cost much less and be just as beneficial. However, when one has more than simple medical problems happen, go seek Emergency Care.

Include Wisdom to Make Your Health Outcomes Awesome

As the Bible notes, 'wisdom is better than rubies; and all the things that may be desired are not to be compared to it.' **Yes!** Wisdom is forward-thinking about what to do or not do when a specific situation arises. Pay attention to wisdom! Further, when action is needed and the proper course is taken, wisdom is the correct recommendation for what to do.

Knowledge in that context is highly desirable. Common sense applications of what to do in the rest of life's situations may not apply to health and wellness issues. We will see.

Assuming your truth is what you want it to be regarding your health is dangerous. Each of us must arrange to live health-providing lives to achieve and retain good health. I made it a standard in my life that if I were to err regarding healthy lifestyle, it would be on the overly cautious side. **Amen! (so be it!)**

Knowledgeable planning for emergencies is invaluable. If your mate or roommate has substantial coronary disease, take a CPR course. Courses are offered locally in most locations.

Whenever sudden severe pain happens, especially in the chest area, abdominal area, or head, call 911. When you have less severe problems but bothersome, depart immediately to get medical care. Don't wait to see if it gets better. If it betters on the way, you can turn around. Know whether or not your doctor has someone on call.

Keep a current document handy of your medical conditions and include a list of medications you are taking and their dosages. Regarding your drugs and supplements, know and take the amount recommended—more is not better and can even be harmful. Know and avoid departures from what is the proper dosing.

We recognize the valuable principle of moderation in life and avoid going overboard in our decisions and actions. Just as you shouldn't spend more than you make, don't eat more than you require nutritionally. These are what we should live by, but often we take in more than we need and risk accumulations that our bodies can't handle.

Don't make the mistake of choosing just to live longer. You also, even more so, want to live better as you live longer. Better realy is BETTER!

Again, assuming truth is what you want it to be is inherently dangerous. Couple that with the "ignore it, and it will go away" mindset and it becomes beset with danger. This is especially true of vascular conditions, including heart attacks and strokes. A beginning heart attack may mimic gastrointestinal upsets, leading one to the bathroom for self-treatment.

The bathroom is one of the most common rooms to be the place of passing on; **be aware**. Severe nausea or gas-type pains can happen early. Vascular problems occur instantly. One minute everything is copacetic, and in the next one, condition appears quite serious.

Is Genetic Predetermination Our Health Causation?

We used to believe that our genes determined all of our health. Some incorrectly continue to blame their genes. **Big mistake!** It proposes that my life and health are not determined by my lifestyle, and I need more medicine to provide a safety net when I get sick.

Now we know otherwise: how you live, how you arrange your lifestyle, is the real foundation of your health (or lack thereof) and it plays a far greater role than your genetic history. A famous Danish study of 2,872 identical twin sets for almost three decades found that our genes' influence on health or disease is actually only 20% to 26%. That means that 74% to 80% of what affects your wellbeing is not genetic. **Wow!**

Multiple other studies show that standard of living benefits accrue no matter what age you start. This dismisses the second great laggard myth: it is too late for a change to benefit me. **Never!** It is never too late; the Jerusalem Longitudinal Cohort Study showed benefits from starting an exercise program even as old as 85 years. You don't have any valid reasons not to act. Get with the program; make it your program.

In other words, you're in the driver's seat. Your behavior determines most of your health and longevity—what I call your "health-span".

Is Your Body Just a Shoddy Living Machine?

A major misconception originated from the consideration of the brain and body as a machine, which as a purely engineering comparison is correct, but although our body obeys mechanical laws, it is structurally biological and only functions mechanically. Machines wear out giving them a mantra: 'Use it and lose it.'

Differently than purely mechanical systems, biological systems constantly repair their wear, cell by cell; cells that die are constantly replaced according to the extent the body determines according to usage. The mantra changes to 'Use it or lose it.' Actually, the more you use it the more you boost its health. **Wow!**

We all know from experience that as we repetitively do something physically or mentally, we become better at it. But this was when I was young—as you age you amend. No, wrong; laws of nature remain the same, whatever your age. You will regain whatever you otherwise would lose by doing; else, there would be no reason for physical therapy and rehab.

This brings us to another health axiom: the secret of health is how much is enough, and the secret of disease is how much is too much. A Chinese proverb exemplifies this point: 'A knife honed to its sharpest will dull soon.' Lifetime health, especially physical, is not a sprint, it is an ultra-marathon. Slow balanced improvement would be best, but one must be careful not to overdo.

This is recommended for those of us who are average; there is no scientific evidence that elite endurance athletes suffer from their extremes.

The important, take-home, lesson of aging is to maintain your quality of life, which should be our goals. Realize your quality of life means being able to do the things you want to do, when you want to do them, granting self-sufficiently.

Run in the park, travel and vacation, garden, manage your affairs, interact with others meaningfully, attend reunions or religious services, go for a night out or to a sporting event, and other activities are the functions of life that give life worth.

Age-Related Disease:
The Real Danger to Wellbeing

As you may have noticed, we are taking the forest-approach to health matters, so we don't get bogged down in details, unless they are essential. Now we will dissect the enemy of health—disease.

Disease is the enemy of wellbeing and can severely limit our functional independence. A Dis-ease meaning a lack of ease is a condition having a host of implications—**all bad**—because disease has potential to reduce wellbeing well below what is normally experienced.

According to Stedman's Medical dictionary, disease produces 'An interruption, cessation, or disorder of bodily function.' Notably, the interval a disease takes from its beginning to when decreases in function occur is very important, as we shall see.

Aging-related diseases are the bad actors: cancer, strokes, heart disease, Alzheimer's, and various others. These are avoidable because they take decades to cause problems! This provides opportunity to remove their causes. Their causes must be abolished to be effective in prevention. YES! Chronic diseases present as illnesses when the body's compensatory mechanisms are trampled.

Doctors treat illnesses correctly by identifying the disease causing it. Advanced diseases are the major basis of disruptions in wellbeing. Medicine's purpose is to restore wellbeing. Headaches are illnesses which can have a dozen different causes, requiring different restorative treatments.

Identifiable signs and symptoms are gauges in diagnosing diseases. A symptom is something a person experiences and a sign is something that can be seen, usually by a doctor. A heart attack is diagnosed by the sudden onset of crushing left frontal chest agony, which tends to radiate down the left arm.

Signs of a heart attack include grasping the left chest, pale countenance, vomiting, and diffuse perspiring. Tests such as an electrocardiogram and blood enzymes confirm the diagnosis. A diagnosis tells the doctor what to do to minimize damage and restore functionality (i.e., health).

Thus, identifiable symptoms and signs define illnesses that result from disease and if the aggregate is unique enough, it satisfies one of the criteria defining a disease. Obvious patterns are termed syndromes. Syndromes often can be named to honor their discoverers, Alzheimer's, the anatomical area affected, myocardial infarction, or the general pathological process, osteoarthritis.

Some have acronyms such as AIDS (Acquired Immune Deficiency Syndrome). There are thousands of syndromes, many of which are unknown outside a particular medical specialty or because they are so rare.

It is important to prepare your body to react favorably in situations that could threaten your health. This defines the core of preventative medicine, but the physician is not in charge. The body's owner is responsible. This is a foundational premise of my health-promoting efforts: You are the occupant and owner of your body. If you accept that fact and give your body the respect it deserves, you will succeed at achieving better health.

Strive to Thrive and Keep Alive: The Vital Keys of Chronic Disease

In medical schools, you might think that the major study emphasis is on disease—not so. The emphasis is on how to diagnose and treat disease which is the correct pathway because medicine's job is to diagnose and treat disease. Those who want to concentrate their study on disease become pathologists. The course in medical school named Pathology is only part of one semester.

In medicine, a witticism went, "Internal medicine doctors know everything and do nothing, surgeons do everything and know nothing, and pathologists know everything and do everything but **too late!**"

When defining the status of health as the ability to function, disease sketchily emerges as a distinct diminishment of functioning. A decline of functioning heralds an illness. Producing pain is a common way the body diminishes one's ability to function. Pain signals that one should rest to allow healing. Another way is generally feeling bad (malaise).

This definition of disease is correct but incomplete, especially considering chronic diseases. Common acute disease's causal agents are most often infectious such as bacteria and viruses. Robert Hooke, an English genius, made one of the most important inventions in determining medical disease causation: the microscope. The microscope is invaluable in diagnosing disease as well, but it diagnoses more because it determines causality.

As an example, high cholesterol does not cause heart disease; it is an "associated factor" termed medically as a risk factor. Lowering cholesterol reduces vascular disease; it does not eliminate the dilemma. The medical literature is chock full of studies showing that elevated cholesterol is a risk factor.

One of the early studies could not be repeated today. Two Finnish mental institutions were assigned a regular diet or a low cholesterol diet for six years and the deaths from heart disease were significantly higher in the regular diet institution. They switched diets and observed for another six years, and the figures reversed. OMG!

There are three recognized criteria to define a disease: 1) a specific causal agent (usually a bacteria or virus); 2) identifiable symptoms and signs; 3) specific anatomical alterations. Any two of these criteria define a disease.

Disease is the most important threat to our health, especially chronic or age-related diseases. To get the most from this book, one must first form a good foundation, based on knowledge of health, disease, metabolism, and medicine.

Look Ahead and Thwart Age-Related Disease Dread

Stress can significantly upsurge age-related (chronic) diseases which are the deadliest threats to health in America. Because of the stress from Covid, chronic disease problems have risen considerably. 70% of all American deaths and 92% of deaths in people over 65 years are from those age-related diseases. Therapeutic cures are directly related to how advanced the disease is when treatment begins, which should emphasize the importance of early recognition. **Be forewarned**!

Early diagnosis superiority emphasizes the need for periodic medical evaluation visits ideally at least twice yearly or even better is quarterly.

I do not want to alarm anyone excessively. Although, I strongly believe that in important matters, if one errs, it should be on the side of carefulness. What I am classifying as alerts are warning signs that possibly indicate manifestations of treatable diseases. It is wise to recognize and scrutinize all alerts your body dispatches.

Note your general wellbeing daily. What is your energy level? Are you feeling more tired lately? Are you requiring more sleep? We all have intermingled good days and bad days but when a pattern of decreasing energy becomes obvious, it indicates a major change in our body. Investigate any change in functioning.

Everyone should weigh himself or herself regularly. Unintended changes in weight are real red flags. Gains and especially unintended losses of over 5% within several months should result in a physician visit. Especially during such times, it is wise to monitor blood pressure. Automatic BP monitors are reasonably priced and easy to use.

Pain is our most common beacon of warning to seek protection by correction. Pain notifies us we have an injury or are being injured and makes us withdraw, and rest the injured part until it has recovered. Pain is unpleasant and teaches us to avoid behavior that could be harmful.

Going to see a doctor for pain is so obvious; you probably wonder why I would mention it. Well, there are several types of pain which are regularly misunderstood as innocent when not. A good example is back pain located in the flanks is likely not spinal; it can be from kidney disease and needs to be checked.

Likewise, upper abdominal pain that radiates to the back often is an abdominal problem, not a back problem. Newly onset back pain (or any pain) that continues for over a week should be evaluated.

Everyone knows heart pain, termed angina, is life-threatening. What they don't know is that in a substantial number, angina is atypical; it may appear as indigestion or jaw pain. In others, about a third, it may be silent. When exerting, if you note extra heartbeats or shortness of breath, get it checked out.

Headaches are another common source of pain. Sudden onset of the worst headache ever should prompt a call to 911. It could signal a weakened artery that is about to rupture. Also, one should become concerned when new recurring headaches begin in older adults, especially if severe enough to suspend daily activities.

Headaches that are brought on with exertion or emotional stress should be investigated. Headaches that are located on one side of the head rather than in general are worrisome.

Let's Collect Our Thoughts About Preventing Blood Clots

I was asked by a friend to explain how an acquaintance had died suddenly from a blood clot. This is overwhelmingly due to blood clots in veins below the waist forming a clot which breaks loose and lodges in the lungs. The name is venous thromboembolism (thrombo=clotting, embolism=traveling). It is an important and often deadly condition.

The number of people having clots form in their legs is estimated at 900,000 per year and the pulmonary embolism results in estimates of up to 100,000 deaths yearly. **Goodness**! The causes were described by one of the most famous physicians of the 19th century; he was Rudolph Virchow (1821 to 1902), a German pathologist.

He described the three predisposing factors: Slowed circulation, increased clotting mechanism, and damage to the lining of the blood vessels. These are to be avoided in as much as possible—it "bees" Clotting Disease's threes.

Slowed circulation is almost certainly the most common causal factor in thrombosis of the veins, most often in the legs. We have two sets of leg veins: superficial which are visible and drain the skin and deep which are not visible and drain the muscles. Clots in the deep veins are the dangerous ones. Inactivity is the principal cause of slowed circulation.

It is another of the remarkable engineering feats of creation design. The heart propels arterial blood, but veins are beyond that propulsion's reach. Instead, the muscles of the legs when contracted squeeze the venous blood during walking and valves keep the blood going backwards during relaxation! Inactivity for prolonged periods such as bed rest slows the circulation, setting the stage for clots; oh no!

Also, a dangerous situation is on long airplane flights. Flights over 4 hours are particularly chancy. I try to briefly walk the isles every hour to be on the safe side. One can also move legs while seated, especially the calf muscles, by raising your heels are far as you can or bringing the knee toward the chest periodically.

Increased clotting can be from genetic or acquired conditions. If one has relatives that have had clots, have clots in unusual places such as the arms, or have repeated clots, they should be evaluated by a physician. Predisposition is in people over 60 years, obesity, recent surgery, or marked dehydration.

Ways you can keep your blood staying thinner is to drink enough water. A good rule of thumb is to drink multiple 8-ounce glasses of liquid daily. YES!

There is a thin layer lining the vessels and heart called endothelium which serves as the Teflon of our bodies. This lining is composed of the only cells that keep blood from clotting. This lining can become damaged as we age and expose tissue that can provoke clotting.

Signals of possible deep vein thrombosis are when one leg or more rarely an arm becomes swollen, tender without cause, or reddened get checked out. **Keep Safe**.

The Miracle of Metabolism: Aging Explained

In the classic movie *City Slickers*, Curley, the trail boss, said it all: 'When it comes to life, there is just one thing,' and he was correct. All living things, including humans, are alive because of the magic of metabolism. You are as healthy and as youthful as your metabolism. As we age, we blame weight gain on our metabolism, which is correct, but our metabolism is much more important than regulating our weight.

As in all things, nothing is inevitable. You can even avoid taxes—if you get elected to congress. Ha. Seriously, you can alter your metabolism.

Metabolism sums the trillions upon trillions of dynamic biochemical reactions continuously taking place every second to keep the body functioning—alive and healthy. These incredible reactions convert food into energy and other incalculable necessary substances allowing life. Cars take us where we want to go because thousands of parts functioning coherently and our bodies are alive because these biochemical reactions make it so.

All these sophisticated processes are divisible into two types of reactions. Reactions involved with breaking down large molecules into smaller ones (catabolism); thereby, producing nutrients for energy or obtaining essential building blocks for future assembly and tissue repair. The second set of reactions is combining the disassembled small molecules to assemble larger ones (anabolism) that is species-specific.

These disassembling and assembling activities include many complex steps that biochemists and molecular biologists spend their careers gradually unraveling. However, it is not necessary to know the steps to understand the process.

Oxygenation resulting in fire is combustion; whereas the process in animal tissue is much more controlled by multiple chemical steps and is termed respiration. Glucose is the principal fuel because it is readily accessible. Besides being taken in with diet, glucose resides in storage tanks in the liver and skeletal muscle—ready on a minute-by-minute basis to be released.

When released, glucose fuel must have an escort to open cellular doors so it can enter cells to provide energy. The escort is insulin, without which the released glucose accumulates in the bloodstream and the resulting disease is diabetes. In non-diabetics as much insulin is secreted as necessary to keep the blood glucose at acceptable levels.

This means consuming more sugar floors the metabolic gas pedal, makes the furnaces run faster, and increases the potentially harmful sparks. These "sparks" are aging molecules.

The total amount of glucose consumed is important for damage to occur, but another consideration applies: the rate at which sugar is absorbed because different foods have different rates of absorption in the bowel of sugars they contain. The fastest rate—i.e., the most harmful absorption—is pure sugar. This is why food products that add extra sugar are bad for your metabolism and your body.

The rate sugar is absorbed from food is important; it is called the glycemic index of food.

You want to limit the aging molecules production by purposefully consuming less sugar and more anti-aging molecules. Anti-aging molecules are in fruits, nuts, and vegetables.

Try Linking Your Thinking to What Will Guarantee That You Foresee a Greater Reality

In order to be successful in any significant endeavor when a good deal of effort is required, one must think carefully and correctly about the situation before taking action. The thinking should be more carefully done depending on the importance of the outcome. Your health and the wellbeing of your body are of primary importance.

Every rational person wants continuing utmost bodily functioning for one's entire lifespan but how to maintain that splendid goal's essence relies on correct thinking about health.

In the material world, everything that produces energy, uses energy or both wears out. And there are rules about those phenomena that determine the rapidity of the wearing out. Think of your automobile and how much it's continued normal functioning depends on your providing adequate maintenance and correct driving habits. Your body is the same.

Aging is necessarily the greatest cause of functional impairment to health. Aside from infections and sudden injuries, the wearing out of our bodies is so slow as to be imperceptible but the damage is cumulative day after day. Our cells ever so gradually change. If you have any doubts, take a look at a photo of yourself from long ago. I just did from 50 years ago when I was in the Navy. OMG!

Just imagine, if cigarette smoking resulted in lung cancer within a month or even within a year, cigarette would have been blacklisted before becoming popular. Smoking would definitely not have continued for 7,000 years. No!

We are programmed from cave dweller times to stuff ourselves because food was scarce and to eat as much high caloric foods as we could was for survival. Now food is constantly available but our brain continues to say stuff yourself. Likewise, our tastes tell us to selectively consume fats and sugary foods because they are high in calories; hence cave dwellers who liked fats would have survived better.

This preference to eat more than needed and prefer fatty foods has led to over 60% of Americans being overweight! And over 40% being severely overweight or obese. Being overweight causes one's body to produce chemicals that speed up the aging process very gradually and ushers in the diseases of aging including cancer, heart disease, stroke, and others that disable or cause demise.

Tailor your diet to not consume potentially harmful foods and instead, develop a taste for foods that contain substances that neutralize the harmful ones produced by your bodies' cells. Learn to enjoy fruits, especially those named berries, and green leafy veggies.

My bride and I have gradually reduced the size of our meals. We almost never finish a restaurant meal. We split it or get a takeout box to go or both. It sure is nice to cut your eating out expense or enjoy another delicious takeout meal at home!

The WHO defines health as, 'Physical, mental, and social well-being, not merely the absence of disease and infirmity.' I want as much of that as I can make happen. Amen!

Be Wise, Energize and Realize the Exercise Prize

Back two and a half millennia, Hippocrates, the father of medicine, noted, 'Walking is man's best medicine'; ever since, all evidence, subjective, empirical, and rigidly scientific, strongly, without exception, have supported that contention. Exercise is not a dirty word; it is very positive. The Merriam Webster dictionary's definition is, 'physical activity that is done in order to become stronger and healthier.' So, exercise is activity with a worthy purpose.

Animals are constructed to be mobile, unlike plants whose job is to be biological solar panels, animals need to forage for fuel. Until the arrival of agriculture and animal husbandry, our hominoid ancestors had to be physically active in acquiring food. Except for certain times of year and certain choice locations, those who caught more game ate more and had increased survival, likely because they traveled greater distances foraging. Now human's greatest foraging problem is standing in line at the checkout stand. **Weekends oh no!**

Everyone knows exercise is beneficial, yet studies show that only one-third of Americans declare that they exercise regularly. And since the exercise duration in the quoted study was only 10 minutes or more, probably half of those do not exercise with enough vigor or long enough to secure health benefits. Error in surveys that ask whether one does something desirable is usually skewed upward with people claiming desired behaviors they do not actually do.

Definite exercise benefits are seen when people moderately exercise for 30 minutes five times a week. **Get your benefits.**

The rewards of physical activity are manifold including the right away and future paybacks. Especially now when we are in such annoying times a 30-minute walk has been shown to be as calming as a tranquilizer! **Take one today!** Regular exercisers not only live longer, but they also live better.

Aging is not a four-letter word; it is mandatorily essential. People gain certain functions growing older but other functions diminish. People in their 40s cannot run as fast as they could in their 20s, and so on. Regular exercise allows retention of our treasured functioning. **Yes, hang on**!

Regular exercise is the best investment one can make toward a restorative future. It not only allows enhanced living in the NOW; it reduces the chance the bad actors of health including heart attack, stroke, and cancer will visit. Suspensions of bad stuff foretell exercise's wholesome effects on the overall aging process.

Aging is molecular damage to one's living cells from "aging molecules" called among other terms "free radicals". They are produced by cells metabolizing to stay alive.

The faster cells produce energy, the more "aging molecules" they produce. Thus, exercise should worsen things, but the body has a wonderful protective mechanism to produce "antiaging molecules" which neutralizes the bad molecules. **Take that bad stuff away!**

Because of exercising's overproduction of protective molecules, exercisers have less loss of function as they continue maturing. You can gain and retain better overall physical and mental performance. **Yeah,** start slow and see your doc if necessary.

Make Your Foundation an Obligation for Socialization

Humans are undoubtedly the most social creatures on the planet, except maybe bees. It is the method we employ to attain—meaning.

According to Professor Robert Nozick, from Harvard, one of the great modern philosophers, meaning by definition, requires crossing boundaries of other sentient beings (i.e., involving others). Love is generally considered the most important attainment, but it is but a subset of achieving meaning and "love" that is without meaning is a worthless endeavor.

A person can care enough for another to say they love them, but the importance of "love" as philosopher Spinoza opined depends on meaning being given to the loved one. Amen!

One is the Loneliest Number was a hit song by the Three Dog Night in 1969. By all available scientific data, the song is accurate. Recent multiple well-done studies have shown social integration has a significant benefit on health. In the Swedish Kungsholmen Project, social integration lengthened useful life even in those over 75 years of age.

In a subset of the Kungsholmen study, over 1200 elderly subjects who had good mental function when the study began, Later 14% developed dementia. Establishing a good social network reduces the chance of the dreaded dementia by 60%. It deposits cash in your mental bank. **Mental cash is good**.

Resilience is a personality characteristic that strongly promotes longevity. Being able to roll with the punches of life is important in reducing the harmful stress life imposes. Support from others, friends in particular, is remarkably stressed busting and friends are created and retained by socialization.

Some of the unhappiest people I have encountered are those who believe life has been unfair to them; life is a stage, a medium for us to act our parts and at best learn. To expect rewards and punishments in harmony with how good or bad we consider our behavior is manifestly absurd. As Shakespeare had Hamlet so ably observe, 'For there is nothing either good or bad, but thinking makes it so.' **Amen!**

Appreciation of those you surround yourself with is important. How many of us wish we had voiced more appreciation to those departed we care for more often? Don't continue that mistake; actively appreciate your friends and loved ones, especially those you have chosen as partners in life. Genuine appreciation is a coin of great value with two sides—contentment for the recipient and giver as well. Like an echo, kind words come back.

The Bible instructs, 'A man that hath friends must show himself friendly (Proverbs 18:24).' Attentiveness, responsiveness, approachable, outgoing, and social are synonyms of friendly.

If you want to be liked by others, sow each relationship's soil with kindness. Kindnesses are especially effective when they are a surprise. Every once in a while, when I am down, I drive to Starbucks, order a double espresso, and hand an extra $10 for the next patron's coffee. My mood elevates from just imagining how that simple gesture makes someone else feel. Unanticipated kindnesses are even more rewarding when given to a friend.

Acquire an Extraordinary Vocabulary

A lifestyle improvisation I have employed throughout my adult lifetime is to ferret out areas of experience that are vital but are considered secondary and just exist on their own without requiring attention. These issues once identified are fully evaluated and a determination made that whether they can be improved and if so, would one's personal standard of living be significantly enhanced? Certainly, one such area is our personal vocabularies. Words initiate and portray our realities.

Our beginning vocabularies of English words were brought to England during the 5th to 7th centuries from Western Germany by Anglo-Saxon immigrants displacing Celtic languages in use. **Wow!** That part of the English lexicon is known today as Old English because it underwent substantial revamping when the Normans conquered Britain in 1071 AD.

Words are the magical illuminators of our very thought realms. They cheer up, clarify, circumscribe, comfort, and even coerce depending on choice of words and intonation. Vocabulary can be used to estimate the intelligence of persons by listeners and readers, and consequently indicates the merit of individuals.

Candidates for jobs, admission to organizations and esteem of associate's level of lexicon differentiates. Thus, it seems that enhancing one's vocabulary is a worthwhile pursuit. **Indeed!**

When listening, or especially when reading, paying close attention to the words is crucial. Eagerly look for new words that you do not understand fully and make a note of them. I have a list of many pages of such findings accumulated over years. Included are words that were recognized but of which, I was not fully certain and included were particularly meaningful words that I don't usually utilize.

An easy and significant system to supplement your vocabulary is to subscribe to a "Word of the Day" site. Merriam-Webster is excellent as are several others to feature an interesting useful word fully defined just pops up in your email.

The vocabulary enhancement process requires that a dictionary be handy to obtain the precise definitions of newly found words. Like everyone, I have copies of the standard bound book dictionaries handy. However, modern technology provides easier and much more efficient means of finding definitions.

An especially helpful source is a website named "One Look Dictionary" which is certainly true to its name because when the word is entered many top dictionaries offer definitions.

Utilizing a thesaurus when accessing new words is helpful in visualizing shades of meaning between similar words. The One Look Site has lists of similar words available with the push of a computer key.

Flashcards are a souped-up approach to jump-starting vocabulary acquiring for those so inclined with the intellectual aptitude and forbearance, but is not for everyone. In choosing that approach, start slowly with a few cards and gradually add more to fit your tolerance so as not to strain your memory capacity.

A further enhancement to memory of new words is to know their etymology. Vocabulary as a "list of words with understanding of their meanings" comes into the English language in the early 1500s from the Medieval Latin word vocabularium "a list of words", from Latin vocabulum "word" which derived from vocare "to name or to call".

Reassess to Possess and
Bless Cheerfulness

These Covid times and there will be others are indeed perturbing times, such as one faces once in a lifetime, but we must avoid embracing self-pity. Self-pity is generally referred to as having a pity party. Those happenings beat the crap out of happiness. When I was an intern at the esteemed Philadelphia General Hospital, now closed, one of my monthly jobs was to collect blood from prisoners at the state prison.

Prisoners would lie down on cots on a basketball court to donate blood and receive $5. Loud b-bop-a-lu-la music blasted in the background. I would go from one cot to others inserting needles and assistants would collect the blood. One day, the guards had machine guns rather than clubs. I asked, 'What is going on?'

'These are the worst of the worst,' a guard replied. 'They will only go out of here in a box.'

I passed down the aisle inserting needles and, yes, I was glad they were locked up. Then I approached an inmate with a big "Howdy Doody" smile. 'You seem extraordinarily happy,' I said.

Convict replied, 'Doc, here I am lying flat on my back in the middle of the day, listenin to good music, and makin five dollars. **Hell, I got it made!**' For more than a half century, when I feel a pity party coming on, I remember that moment and think or if I am alone shout, **'Hell, I got it made'** and everything straightens out.

Sporadically, there is a clustering barrage of unpleasant info, much of which is pap titled as news. One should limit exposure to unpleasant news. I hardly watch or listen to the news anymore because it is easy to overdose. News rarely reports the millions of good self-sacrificing events because humans apparently are fascinated by tragedy much more than everyday good deeds. Otherwise, with wrecks, rubbernecking would not be a universal practice on highways.

Regret is an emotion arising when we could have acted differently and avoided an unfortunate outcome. It is reliving a bad time with guilt superimposed. It is traveling through life looking through a rear-view mirror.not wise. We need to learn from our mistakes and then travel onward without suffering guilt by revisiting regretful situations.

If one learns from his or her past, the undesirable past must be closed as a meaningful experience and does not need to be relived.

One of the principal venues for happiness is to look where there is meaning. Meaning according to a modern philosopher, Robert Nozick, requires communication with other intelligent beings. As mentioned, but worth repeating, the most valuable painting in the world according to Guinness World Records is the Mona Lisa.

It is insured for over a half billion dollars. It has a great deal of meaning in addition to its value. But if it were preserved in a locked vault where no one could appreciate it, it would retain value but lose meaning. **Yes**! Appreciate your meanings and incentivize to add more.

I had a good, remarkably resilient, Jewish friend who when disappointed, would shrug and say, 'This too will pass.' **And it will!**

Making Your Home a True Safe Harbor

Personal households are generally considered one's safe harbor but surprisingly, homes provide the settings for substantial accidents. 60% of unintended injuries happen at one's home! OMG! Perhaps this is because we spend more time there than any other dwelling.

Many falls at home are serious, with over 800,000 injured yearly requiring hospitalizations and with almost 40,000 deaths from head injuries and bone fractures. OMG 2! Besides falls, burns and poisonings occur too frequently in homes. I'm not saying your home is entirely unsafe; I'm telling you it can and should be made safer.

Be certain that sturdy handrails are on all stairways. Have motion sensor night lights in areas with diminished lighting and areas where people might need to go at night. Hallways and spaces where lighting is diminished should definitely be included. Throw rugs should have non-slip under liners or tape or be removed.

Non-slip waxes for wood floors are readily available and do not need to be applied often. Replace any unstable furniture and have chairs with steadfast arms to assist sitting and standing.

More serious injuries can occur when falls occur because of tripping on pets, especially dogs. Thus, be extra careful around pets when erect and moving about. Never step over pets, even smaller animals. They can suddenly move under foot. Watch carefully to keep pet's toys from being left in walkways.

In rooms having shelves, especially the kitchen, move all regularly used items to the lower shelves no higher than eye level for easy visual accessibility. This will limit standing on footstools and the associated chance of falling.

The bathroom and other areas where water could accumulate are higher risk areas, especially the shower. Statistics disclose that 80% of falls occur in the bathroom. **Wow!** Place non-slip floor coverings in areas where water could accumulate on the floors. In the shower, place non-slip floor mats, or do as we did and have a slip resistant pebble mosaic floor installed. With that even when feet are copiously covered with soap, one cannot forcefully cause their feet to slip.

Install a grab bar or bars depending on the shower's configuration inside the shower and outside close to where you will towel dry. Also, place a plastic non-slip mat in the bathtub. And, as mentioned, put a stable mat or mats where one can get into and out of the bathtub.

Burns and scalds are other means of unintentional household injuries which are avoidable by planning forward. Mount and maintain household fire alarms and formulate a general plan of escape if they go off. Periodically examine exposed electrical wiring and replace any that is threadbare.

Set your hot water tank temperature to 120 degrees. Burns are rapid at higher temperatures. 6 seconds will scald at 140F and 30 seconds at 130F but temperatures at 120F will take 5 minutes! **Keep safe**. Turn all stove pots and pans handles to the side. If you have a fireplace, have an expert inspect it every five years or any time you see a change. When burned immediately, place the injured flesh under cold water.

Further, I consider my body the house for my mind and exercise frequently along with daily balance exercises. Consider choosing a comfortable chair and sit and stand repeatedly.

Promotion of Emotion Has the Ability to Enhance Stability

There is considerable scientific information that maintaining a positive approach to life has many health benefits. **Positive is best.** Positive people live longer and lead healthier lives. Individuals with positive outlooks are troubled by fewer chronic diseases, less depression or anxiety than those with a negative outlook.

Approach to life, and attitude about it, is tinted or even established by our emotions. And guess what, we can manage what emotions we are feeling. Our bodies react to an amazing extent to our emotional stance. Stress and the long-term detriment it brings from stress hormones is lessened with our emotions.

Stress hormones are released in response in response to bothersome moods. They prepare our bodies for a fight or flight response raising alertness, tightening muscles, and raising blood pressure which is without problems if occurring only occasionally but detrimental when overdone.

There is little meaning discoverable in life without emotions, but few have made efforts to define them let alone how to improve them and especially how to keep emotions rational. There are almost boundless numbers of emotions because there are virtually limitless ways, we may feel about what we encounter or contemplate. However, Paul Ekman, a noted psychologist, identified six basic emotions: anger, disgust, fear, happiness, sadness, and surprise.

In my opinion, the emotion that gives the most positive uplift to mood is **gratitude**.

What characterizes the different emotions? William James stated that anger represents slights, fear represents dangers, shame represents failures to live up to an ego ideal, sadness represents losses, happiness represents progress toward goal achievement, pride represents enhancement of one's ego identity. Indeed!

Naturally, emotions are part of one's humanity and are necessary, but they must be controlled. It must be remembered that we have a conscious and an unconscious self to control. The James-Lange psychological theory proposes that the conscious self is informed about what to feel emotionally by physical actions; we frown or cry and begin to feel sad or we smile or laugh and feel happy.

Our conscious brain can take charge to smile and laugh more often. Also, start to frown less and to resolve not to get angry without thinking whether anger is worth of the cost to your wellbeing. There!

A great deal of damage can be the result of extremes of emotion, and it is best to decide to control the two chief emotions: anger and happiness. Surplus happiness can spiral into euphoria that can result in behaviors that humiliate. Even worse, anger can spiral out of control into frenzied rage and even if one is alone, non-reconcilable behaviors can emerge. Moderation!

Maintain a happy countenance and you will look better and younger. In a study, subjects were asked to estimate the age and emotional state of pictures in groups of the same people either smiling or frowning. Subjects so tested considered smilers were more likable and younger to a significant extent. OMG!

When you feel an emotion erupting, make it a practice to hesitate and consider what it really means and what your reaction should be in response. Anger hurts the angry person because stress hormones are released. I have simply developed a "so what the heck" attitude in all cases unless my health or a loved one's health is threatened, and that is extremely rare.

Don't Flop, Stop,
Think, and Then Act

In my 40s, I took up scuba diving. I'd always wanted to experience the sensation of being nearly weightless underwater, gliding along, breathing naturally, and observing marine life up close. I'm sure I've forgotten much of what the then-young instructor had told us about how to defog a mask or properly clean a wetsuit.

But what I will never forget is what he said that first day—and this was before we even got wet. 'Divers!' He barked. 'Obey the rules or death is minutes away.'

That stuck with me. He went on, his voice an octave higher, making sure he had all of us with him. 'If there is anything to remember it is this: Stop! Think! Then act! It is the most important rule in scuba diving. It one day might save your life.'

Good health is largely achievable by following the same advice. (And, just like diving, ignoring the rules about your health can bring about your departure much sooner.) Following the rules saved my life both when diving and from a heart attack.

When in Palau (a group of isolated great for diving islands in the South Pacific), I dove a multi-chambered cave named the Chandelier. My guide and I went into the cave, as a group of inexperienced oriental divers exited. They stirred the sediment, a real no-no in cave diving, so visibility became so bad that I lost track of my guide who kept swimming onward.

Soon, I could no longer hear my guide; I was alone in the darkness. I stopped, thought, and then acted. The guide was very experienced so he must have swum directly to an opening in the chamber that led to the outside. I noted the reading of my depth gauge and angle of ascent and kept to the same route. To proceed otherwise may have taken me into a wrong chamber.

I surfaced in the correct chamber, took off my mask, and the local guide blurted, 'Where you beeeen?'

Danger is so apparent in SCUBA diving; death's bony finger is clearly visible. Death's bony finger is just as clear in our unhealthy lifestyles, but we often choose to ignore warnings. We must be in denial. We consider ourselves exempt from the statistics that declare: if you embrace unhealthy behaviors, you will suffer.

I was billeted at a Marine Corps base during the Viet Nam War and 58,220 brave soldiers who hoped they were invincible died. No one is invincible. Threats apply to us all equally. It obviously does, but why should it really matter whether the actual dying takes a few minutes or several decades?

Remember, also, suffering in one instance is a few minutes, compared possibly to months in the other. Without healthy living, one is drowning over a twenty-year period.

In England, the government has a healthy lifestyle program it offers to people at high-risk for cardiovascular disease with dismal results. One-third decline to enroll, 40% refused screening, 70% sporadically attend, and high dropout rates complete the picture. Goodness! Why is non-compliance a serious problem? Stop, think, and then act—long-term for a greatly improved life and life expectancy.

59

The Essentials About Essential Hypertension

Hypertension is truly the silent killer. It is the most common chronic disease accelerator in people over 65 years. Everyone knows high blood pressure can be harmful but actions to manage it properly are not generally appreciated. Overall, one of three adults has hypertension this climbs to two of three in those over 65 years.

Twenty percent of hypertensives do not know they have a problem and about 40% with hypertension are not being treated. More alarming is the fact that even though highly effective treatment is available only one-third of those with hypertension are adequately controlled.

Hypertension pounds the blood vessels and is widely known to increase vascular disease, especially strokes. Hypertension is a major contributor to dementia, especially the dreaded Alzheimer's disease. Since there are no curative treatments for Alzheimer's disease, prevention is the only strategy.

Such dismal results in treating hypertension indicate something is wrong with the process of therapy for hypertension. Actually, hypertension's suboptimal management is a superb example of why patient participation in personal health maintenance is necessary. And why basic health knowledge is essential to adequately participate.

A number of effective classes of medicines for hypertension are available. Medications can be switched when not working and often are combined with other meds to achieve desired results. Find a physician with sufficient knowledge as to which meds to use in your particular case.

But the much more common problem is inadequate monitoring and follow-up. Sporadic medical appointments provide a snapshot of what is a dynamic health problem. Blood pressure varies according to the activity, mental state, and time of day. Usually, a single blood pressure recording each visit is used to determine therapy and unless the pressure is markedly elevated, follow-up recordings with reevaluation can be repeated in weeks or months.

Let's examine the essentials for improved hypertension therapy. In over 90% of hypertension, the cause is unknown to medical science—called essential hypertension, thus the title of this probe.

Overfilling the vascular system is a known cause of high blood pressure. Salt keeps water in the body and in excess overfills the system. If you drink a quart of pure water, your kidneys will excrete the excess within an hour. Lace the water with 1% salt and it will take a day for the kidneys to excrete the excess. Keep salt intake to a minimum!

Those having hypertension and those over 65 should periodically (at least weekly) take their pressures at home. There are accurate automatic blood pressure monitors available for less than $100 and are good investments.

Omron 10 series is a machine that is highly regarded. Your physician can help you check your monitor's accurateness.

At a regular time, each week, apart from stressful activities, in the middle of the day (BP tends downward in the evening), sit for 5 minutes and then take your blood pressure, several times. Do not measure pressure just after exertion or drinking caffeinated beverages. You can easily defeat the silent killer.

Weighing in on the Subject of Weight: How Much is Too Much

The weight management subject will require a series of missives to deliver. This, the first is when to recognize you have something that should weigh on you.

This subject may not be popular in the USA, especially in those more senior but like taxes, it must be dealt with properly or the consequences can be catastrophic. Most people are in denial believing that weight gain just is inevitable in senior hood. **Not so.** My grandparents and mom were in rest homes and there were almost no residents that were obese.

The main number for weight determination that you should calculate is your BMI (Body Mass Index). Google "BMI calculation" input the info about your height and weight and a number will appear. 25 or less and you are OK. Over 30 is obese and schedules a bumpy ride! Get with the program! Healthier living requires recognizing the truth and acting sensibly.

Waist circumference is another way to determine whether action is needed. Women should be concerned over

35 inches and men over 40 inches. If, when standing straight, you cannot see your toes, your belly needs attention. Another perhaps more meaningful measurement is the waist circumference to height ratio. It should be 50% or less.

Where you have stored fat is important. Generalized subcutaneous fat is less harmful than "visceral adiposity" which is a kind way to announce someone has a "beer belly". A greatly increased abdominal size is a factor in the undesirable metabolic syndrome which is to be avoided as it forebears' health problems.

Our bodies have the capacity to store energy in the form of adipose tissue which is the polite way of saying fat. This was necessary because our ancient hunter ancestors were opportunistic eaters with a real danger of starvation.

Hunters might be successful with a kill and provide a feast only afterward not have food for an extended period. Those who gorged themselves and their bodies preserved the excess survived periods in which others perished. We have their genes and therefore their appetites.

In modern times, when immoderations are everywhere present, excessive gorging can overwhelm the subcutaneous storage spaces and result in our important organs becoming fat containers. The most obvious are abdominal organs with the essential organs liver and pancreas being the first ones to suffer.

Our bodies do not make more cells to store fat as more fat accumulates. The storage cells for fat enlarge. Capillaries furnishing oxygen for energy needed for life do not increase and diffusion is limited, so big fat cells can become depleted of energy from lacking oxygen and signal they need help.

Cells that are distended secrete signaling materials termed cytokines (from Greek meaning cell motion). These can start the body to make preparations for removing cells that will increase the aging process. You do not want this. Aging does not need to be speeded up! Most everyone would like to decelerate the aging process.

Are We Really What We Eat?
Yup, We Sure Are

We find comfort when thinking we are identical to our cars and other property, assuming that we take in the things we need and use them like fuel or building materials, independently from the "US". But not so fast, what we consume becomes part and parcel of our very bodies; the stuff we consume becomes the stuff that is us. Two of the three major nutrients (fats and sugars) produce only energy (or become stuffing for our fat cells).

They keep us alive but do not become the substance of us. Protein on the other hand constitutes the bricks and mortar of our bodies.

The minimal protein daily requirement (MDR) presently recommended by authorities is 0.8 grams for every kilogram of body weight or about 60 grams for an average sized male adult. It is about 10% less for females. For comparison, a nickel by law weighs 5 grams (not a lot).

There is considerable concern that the MDR for protein is insufficient for the elderly. The reasoning is that muscle loss occurs as we age, and a healthier body has more muscle and less fat which is the opposite of what nature imposes.

Nature imposes a gradual loss of muscle mass (sarcopenia) as we age because of decreased hormones and decreased physical activity. This combination contributes to reduction in physical ability and decreased metabolism (BMR). The decrease in metabolism contributes to increase in body fat which always means increased aging with all its associated problems, including speeded demise.

One authority noted that increased protein intake was associated with increased muscle mass and longer survival. He proposed that the MDR for protein be doubled in individuals over 65 years. Wouldn't you like to look younger?

So, maximum muscle synthesis is what we all desire. No, I know we don't wish to compete in body building contests with the likes of the "Arnold Schwarzenegger's" but we would like to keep our physiques from going south. This can be altered for your benefit function and appearance. **Better** is always superior.

Some studies show that not only the amount but the timing is important. One study stated older adults taking in 30 grams of protein with each meal was optimal. Doubling the protein intake to 1.6 grams per kilogram body weight over 10 weeks substantially increased lean body mass and increased leg strength.

A leaner body mass moves the BMR (the resting rate at which your body consumes calories) in an optimistic direction, every added pound of muscle daily removes 60 additional calories, without you doing anything. Also, increased leg strength reduces the chance that you will fall. And, in addition, more muscle increases your functionality.

The ability to live well is determined by being able to do not what you need to do but moreover being able to do what you want to do and being more confident about living soundly. AMEN!

Dieting is Not a
Four-Letter Word

Healthy diets abound but for rock-solid dependability, we should trust the two most studied geographically named diets: the Mediterranean Diet and the Okinawan Diet. Located thousands of miles apart with vastly different cultures, they are among the longest-lived and healthiest people on earth.

The Mediterranean diet is primarily the diet of southern Italy and people living in the south of Italy live longer than northerners do. Okinawa is a southern Japanese island, and the Okinawans live longer than other Japanese. These statistics are particularly impressive when one considers that the Italians (at #4) and Japanese (on top at #1) are nations having the highest national personal longevities on Earth.

There is nothing wrong with adopting a "named" diet but most in need find that drastically altering their eating intake is difficult. My approach is to expand foundational knowledge about a subject and let people design what makes sense to them.

Foodstuffs are commonly classed in three general categories: fat, carbohydrates (sugars), and proteins. For weight control, calories are all important not the volume. Calories are depicted by calories per gram (a nickel is 5 grams, pretty darn small): fat is 9, carbs are 4 and protein is 4. However, the expenditure of our body's transformation of the foodstuffs into calories varies.

Fat conversion into energy costs only 3% and sugar's loss is negligible. Apparently, protein was not intended by nature to be used for energy. Transformation of it wastes 30%, so a gram of protein releases a meager 2.8 calories per gram. **Yea!**

Consuming more protein has other advantageous results: protein is more filling than the others, by far. It increases awareness and that possibly is the result of its Specific Dynamic Action. SDA is an increase in metabolism of about 25% for several hours after a meal. This lowers the caloric intake by even more! SDA was described for at least 70 years and is known by very few. Amazing!

What about the standard three meals a day which are entrenched into present thinking? In ancient times, there was often not even one meal a day depending largely on food availability. Romans ate one meal daily and considered consuming more meals gluttony. Lunch showed up as "nuncheon", an old Anglo-Saxon word which meant a quick snack. It was not regularly practiced until the 19th century.

The timing of meals makes a difference. Our bodies operate according to a "Circadian (daily) Rhythm" because of the alterations of a 24-hour day with hormone induced sleep-wakefulness cycles. Simply remember the last jet lag you experienced!

Eating a late lunch can cause a weight problem. One study showed that women who ate their major meal as breakfast rather than dinner lost weight. One of the strongest associations of meal timing and weight gain was a study examining the time between the last meal of the day and timing of sleep. So, it appears that we should logically try to eat the most food earlier in the day.

Weight Self-control by Limiting Your Pie-Hole's Food Patrol

Any worthwhile endeavor starts with several possible actions to achieve the desired goal. Success is achieved by choosing the spot-on approach and having the resolve to see it to completion. Both the ideation and actions require an understanding of the logic behind the ideal way. The Bible in Proverbs 5 states this truth as "Get wisdom, get understanding".

Two entities establish our material world: pure energy and material energy. Each can under the right circumstances be converted to the other; this conversion is what makes the universe operate and keeps us alive. The living tissue of our bodies is converted to energy that allows us to move about and we fuel up by consuming material energy.

Our body weights clearly are determined by how much fuel we take in. If we take in more energy than we utilize, we gain weight which is stored as fat tissue. Likewise, fat is released into the bloodstream and used as reserve energy when needed. Fat cells size depends on how much energy (fat) we have stored in them, little fuel storage tanks if you will. Little is better.

There are three principal types of bodily fuel: fats, sugars, and protein. Fat is high octane, sugar is medium octane, and protein is low octane. Sugar is absorbed immediately and pushed inside cells. As blood sugar rises, it turns off fat metabolism and causes fat to be stored as lipid in fat cells. Thus, it has a dual physiologic mechanism for increasing body fat. **Oh no.**

Fats are high octane containing 9 calories per gram and just like sugars converted to energy easily. Once again, a nickel weighs 5 grams for perspective.

Protein starts with less than half the calories as fat and is intended to be building blocks for our bodies, and if not needed, it must be converted to energy and loses ten times as much energy in the conversion to energy step as fat's consumption, about 30% and thus it provides only 2.8 calories per gram. Thus, high protein foods reduce calorie intake considerably. Yea, protein is good for weight control.

Plus, a high protein meal speeds up metabolism for hours afterwards; termed the "specific dynamic action". High protein meals will promote weight loss, especially at breakfast when the increased metabolic rate from the protein will boost the daily activities increase and help shrink your fat. All meats have protein but choose lean cuts.

Our bodies have two selves the conscious and the subconscious. The subconscious tells the awake self when they are satisfied with the amount eaten. We might think we are full when the stomach is distended but moreover, fullness can be with the duration and effort spent consuming the meal.

Start to establish fullness control by using smaller plates and plating reduced amounts. Make the process gradual for the top result with the least irritation. This will aid in the steps to adjust your subconscious sell's appetite. Reduce the size of your bites and you will get a tastier meal and be satisfied sooner.

I have adjusted to get at least ten bites when eating a cookie. Yum! Continue to chew longer making each bite last and provide more satisfaction than in hurried eating would offer.

The Format to Combat Fat

No doubt, fat is one of the more unpleasant words in the English language. Fat cells are of two types: white fat (to store energy, more) and brown fat (baby fat, to create warmth, fewer). In numbers, they only make up less than 1% of the body's total cells (at 25 billion of 30 trillion total cells) but there appears to be many more because as one gains fat the cells enlarge; fat cells do not appreciably multiply!

This is an aging and sickness-promoting problem because as fat cells expand the capillaries feeding them oxygen don't grow becoming inadequate and the deprived cells signal that they are in trouble. These signaling substances increase the bodies aging process as the enlarged cells pepper the body with damaging substances.

Some of the damaging substances increase the body's inflammatory status with many long-term effects, including increased cancer, vascular disease, dementia, and arthritis among others. Following fat reduction, markers for inflammation decreased.

So, how can we best reduce our body's fat load and become healthier? The majority of calories are contained in fat (9/gram), next sugars (4/gram), and last in protein

(4/gram but actually 2.8/gram). Most diets (not a dirty word) concentrate on calories which seems the right approach for weight loss.

However, Hall researched the subject in an interesting way and found that more fat was lost by restricting fat than low-carb diets when the same calorie restrictions applied. There should be no surprise there. Overall weight loss does not vary between the two restricted diets, but the low fat diet reduced more fat.

Exercise is hyped for weight and fat loss. Some important facts should be appreciated to maximize efforts. Our bodies have three main energy sources: immediate, reserve, and supplemental. The immediate is composed of blood sugar complexes, located in the liver and muscle to provide rapid sources of energy. The reserve source is fat, naturally in our fat cells, released when needed.

The supplemental is our muscular protein which is converted into sugar in the liver when the other two sources are insufficient. Muscle breakdown happens during starvation and is appreciated as wasting away of body mass.

There is evidence that calorie-restricted diets that include added protein do more to reduce body fat. Further and perhaps more important, when the metabolic indicators predicting future heart disease were measured, combining calorie-restricted and high protein diets provided the best improvement of the associated danger.

This means that for the first 30 minutes or so during sustained exercise, the body principally uses its stored sugar and after 30 minutes begins to call upon the fat cells. Then one can be hungry just after exercise and want to take in calories, defeating any significant reduction in fat.

Accordingly, for fat reduction exercise longer. Resistance training can work well if muscle is increased.

Remember when you were young, you could eat anything you wanted without appreciable weight gain. Lean body mass burns the calories up.

Appreciate That it is Great to Hydrate

As we age, our instinctive regulatory mechanisms can become a little disordered, and we may not become appropriately thirsty as needed. Also, older people's fluid reserves shrivel. This is why dehydration is more common as you age. But one may think: All of my life, my body has told me when to drink, and I have done just fine. **Rethink that now.** There are studies documenting that as many as one out of every four seniors is dehydrated.

There are several undesirable effects in chronically dehydrated seniors including earlier mortality. Pneumococcal pneumonia is the deadliest of infectious diseases that trigger over 1.5 million emergency room visits and over 40,000 deaths in America a year. This plague is more common in dehydrated people.

Dehydration is associated with decreased cognitive performance. In one excellent study, in several thousand older participants, scientists measured serum particles to water concentration in the blood and tested mental functioning. In those seniors with undersupplied water, mental functioning shrunk noticeably.

In the case of quantities, the central question is "How much water is enough?" The question is well studied, and recommendations are eight containers of eight ounces of liquid for men and six for women daily. Allow more when engaging in activities involving sweating, GI illness, or when feverish.

Mild dehydration can produce fatigue, headache, light headiness, and dry skin. You are well-hydrated if your mouth has more noticeable saliva than just being moist and when skin snaps back if tweaked. Most importantly, if your urine is clear or only slightly yellowed, it is better. **Check periodically**.

Remembering How to Save Your Memory: Stopping Self-Wither

Let's face it: Mental functioning like physical functioning reaches a high point and a person over 65 years cannot expect to have physical or mental function like they had decades earlier. The normal physical sign of aging is ascribed to diminished gray matter (what you think with) include the frontal lobes where executive functioning (reasoning) takes place, so an aged brain does not work as quickly as before and the hippocampus where recent memory takes place.

Let's face the facts: memories make up the self and you don't want to see your personal self-wither.

In a very thought-provoking study, a researcher used MRI technology to compare the memory centers of the brain in London taxi drivers to London bus drivers. The taxi drivers memory centers were larger and their size was larger the longer they had been driving taxis which emphasizes **use it or lose it!**

The Harvard (pronounced Haaaavdd) Medical website points out that not only age is associated with memory problems, depression, anxiety, stress, and a lack of sleep.

Eliminate any of those causes and you will improve the root cause.

Short term memory decline is the most noticeable and aggravating, by far. I will attempt to offer some compensatory mechanisms to lessen everyday burdens. Short-term memory is defined as super short—up to 30 seconds. Our brains record immediately and decide within 30 seconds whether to keep or forget what we have noted. It does not seem like much but much of our ability to continue independent living depends on short-term memory.

Knowing when you have done something is important, especially taking meds, feeding pets, and turning off the stove, etc.

Much of all and especially senior forgetting is due to failure to properly use our attention. Our concentrating on our attention span decreases as we age. A possible clue to retaining info is shown in a study where subjects were to be given rewards, of either high value or low value. The high value rewards were remembered significantly better than lesser rewards.

It is important to keep valued info in memory and we all could keep a possible date's phone number in our brain intact because it was rated important. Other important info like possible test material stuck with us. **Oh yeah**?

Another possible underlying factor in memory difficulty is your meds: Especially, true for anti-anxiety, cholesterol lowering (statins), narcotics, meds for Parkinsonism, hypertension (beta blockers), and antihistamines. Check with your doctor or pharmacist about the potential of your meds and consider perhaps in stopping temporarily or changing them would pertain.

Doesn't it seem to occur more and more as time passes that a senior goes into a room and forgets why they are there—**GADS?** It is normal because of shriveled focus. The aggravating event markedly diminishes if you focus for a second on why you are going into another room. When going for an object, I get a mental picture of the object sought, such as my keys or wallet or for an action get a mental picture. **O-yea!**

Whenever, I leave the house there are three things I must retrieve: keys, wallet, and sunglasses, in addition to my pants. As I open the garage door, I ask myself, 'do you need to take anything else?' If the something else is needed for an upcoming trip, I place it by my keys. Also upon returning home, my first routine (unless the house is on fire) is to replace the objects taken in their specific spaces.

To remember a specific responsibility for a future obligation or appointment, I employ Mr. Smartphone as a reminder or if the action is later that same day, I may shift my wedding band to the other hand. It works.

Just before bedtime, I have four things to do: Take my ER (extended release) meds (I take meds that allow a single daily dose), setup coffee, get nightly bedside water, and attach my phone to a specific charger. The master bathroom has motion activated night lights which eliminates the chance of accidents.

Certain foods especially those containing flavonoids, have been shown to enhance memory by enhancing nerve cell's connections which are the computer chips of your brain. **Go neurons!** Not only is short-term memory improved, but it is also proposed that flavonoids improve spatial memory as well. Short-term memory allowing independence and spatial memory (where you are located) are, in fact, functions that are first blunted in early dementias.

Flavonoids are available as supplements but there is concern about taking them because when they are excessive harm can result. There is no danger from consuming more fruits and veggies, especially leafy ones, to get more safe flavonoids to supercharge your brain. Berries, nuts, beans, plums, coffee, and tea are especially packed with these good products for brain substances.

There are many supplements for sale that make super claims but offer little scientific support. Aside from prescription meds, the ones which have the greatest likelihood of being helpful to keep your squash intact are vitamin D, Folate, and B12. Deficiencies of vitamin D is associated with accelerated mental decline which is why I recommend it as a supplement for older folks.

There is evidence, though not indisputable, that Folate and B12 have roles in mental preservation. One investigator shed light on the possible confusion. Dr. Tangney measured not only the serum concentration of B12 (which did not correlate with mental status in older adults), he measured the bodies' byproducts of B12 and found their levels did correlate with lower levels having shoddier mental function.

Another large French study supplemented subject's diet with antioxidants and tested for cognitive decline over an 8-year period. Those whose diet was supplemented had preserved mental function. **Take your vits!**

Mnemonic Systems (named for Mnemosyne the Greek goddess of memory) is a system for memorizing multiples of names or facts—those Greeks did it all! The routine involves attaching specific ideas to items in your house in the order they belong and making a mental trip to identify the succession of ideas.

There is a plethora of scientific information documenting a positive correlation (over 4,600 to be exact)—**triumph!** Studies on the effect of remaining physically fit on memory shows real benefits for memory. Even better, the degree of fitness increased the enhancement of mental performance. As previously mentioned, young males were tested for chemical factors that show increased motor function and physical abilities correlated with mentation.

Enrich Your Cerebral Squash, Don't Let it Wither

Specific mental health problems, especially depression, stress, and excess anxiety, can impact memory damagingly as can sleep deprivation. Anyone having these problems can be assured that correction of these glitches will improve memory.

Another correctable underlying aspect is your meds: Especially true for antianxiety meds, cholesterol lowering (statins), narcotics, meds for Parkinsonism, hypertension meds (beta blockers), and antihistamines. Check with your doc or pharmacist about the potential of your meds being at fault and the wisdom in stopping them temporarily or changing them might pertain.

Certain foods especially those containing flavonoids, have been shown to enhance memory by boosting nerve cell's connections which are the computer chips of your brain. Flavonoids are found in fruits (blueberries apples, pears, and bananas), vegetables (onions, tomatoes, bell peppers, and celery), chocolate, and beverages like tea and wine—*laissez le bon temps rouler*!

Not only is short-term memory improved but it is also proposed that flavonoids improve spatial memory (recognizing where you are) as well. You don't want to get lost. Short-term memory allowing independence and spatial memory are, in fact, functions that are blunted foremost in aging and early dementias.

Flavonoids are available as supplements but there is concern about taking them because when they are taken in excess harm can result. There is no danger from consuming more fruits and veggies to get more safe flavonoids to supercharge your brain. Go brain cells.

The small hippocampus (one on each side of the bottom of the brain) are responsible structures for short-term memory and spatial recognition of where you are located. One supplement, resveratrol, has some promise to improve hippocampus function. However, there are many supplements for sale that make super claims but offer little scientific support.

Aside from prescription meds, the ones which have the greatest likelihood of being helpful to keep your squash intact are vitamin D, folate, and B12. Deficiencies of vitamin D is associated with accelerated mental decline which is why I recommend it as a supplement for older folks. More is not better when taking vitamin D. The safe long-term dosage is one thousand international units which sounds like a lot but it is less than a milligram.

There is evidence, though not indisputable, that folate and B12 have roles in mental preservation. One investigator shed light on the possible confusion, Dr. Tangney, measured not only the serum concentration of B12 (which did not correlate with mental status in older adults). He measured the bodies' byproducts of B12 and found their levels did correlate with those with lower levels having shoddier mental function.

Another large French study supplemented subject's diet with antioxidants and tested for cognitive decline over an eight-year period. Those whose diets were supplemented had preserved mental function. Another well-designed study showed that giving supplemental folic acid and B12 to elderly subjects over 24 months in immediate and long-term mental function. **Take your vits!**

Stop Your Aging's Brain Drain: Squash Preservation 101

Remembrance competency is divided generally into long-term, short-term, and working memory. Long-term memory is an enormous collection of memories dating from the immediate to as far back as our brain can take us. Short-term memory keeps us functioning in the now and decides what to store in the permanent category or it's bye-bye.

Working memory is what we do with short-term memory to make decisions as to actions we need to take. In general, short-term memory evaporates first and have no doubts, it is our survival mode! Our working memory uses "shorty" to make decisions which chances being incorrect with limited facts from "shorty".

There is a plethora of scientific information documenting a positive correlation of physical fitness (over 4,600 articles in PubMed to be exact) with wellbeing's mental security. **Triumph!**

Studies on the effect of remaining substantially fit on memory shows real benefits for cognition. Even better, the degree of physical fitness increased the enhancement of mental performance incrementally when young males were tested for chemical factors that indicate increased motor function and physical abilities their mentation was better.

Even more important as we age, is preservation of the part of the brain that processes short-term memory and spatial relations, the hippocampus. It shrinks structurally as we age. **Oh no!** So, our short-term memory dwindles, and it becomes easier to get lost. A small protein, nerve growth factor (BDNF), keeps our brain cells operating better. Unfortunately, this brain health promoting factor decreases as we age.

As mentioned earlier, a small but important portion of the brain, labeled the hippocampus (hippo), allows us to function self-sufficiently; great. Our hippos in elder life shrink a few percentages yearly. Some well-done studies published in reputable journals, showed that adults who joined an exercise program increased their Hippo volumes erasing 1–2 years of shrinkage.

In addition, and just as important, they increased their levels of nerve growth factor (BDNF) which means less overall loss of brain cells from aging. This "brain cell preservation" factor is found to increase after exercise which keeps the mental squash intact. The term neurotrophic stands for neuro=nerve, trophic=promoting cellular growth, differentiation, and survival. **Wow!** That is important stuff.

The indisputable evidence showing the value of BDNF is from a study on several thousand subjects over 65 years that showed a correlation of blood levels with the chance of developing the dreaded Alzheimer's disease (AD) over a ten-year period. Higher levels of BDNF in normal subjects at the studies' start had a 50% reduction of dreaded AD. Yea!

Even more interesting, when subjects were started on moderate exercise programs 3 days a week and had their BDNF measured before and after 12 weeks, the post-exercise levels were significantly higher. There are many, many well done studies verifying the value of physical fitness enhancing mental fitness. Be advised, to see your doc if you have health problems, start slowly, and build up gradually.

Don't Hesitate to Concentrate on Medication Information for Maximum Salvation

Three-fourths of all adults in the US regularly take prescription medicines which are remarkable aids to maintaining healthy lifestyles. When taking these lifesaving components, it is essential for you not to manage them unless you are a health professional. I am, but I always use my doctor's management for my meds without alteration.

Over time, one may decide they want to see about taking fewer meds because they seem to be doing well. Don't do it on your own, especially with meds intended to treat heart problems, cholesterol, blood pressure, or diabetes. Instead, when at appointments for routine checkups, ask if any meds can safely be diminished or discontinued.

Generic medications are medicines not having a brand name because the exclusive rights protection of the parent company expired after 20 years. They are rigorously tested by the FDA to be sure they are identical to branded meds and that they are absorbed the same by the body. **Yes, same**. Since generics average costing one-fifth as much, ask your doctor if they are available and will meet your needs. **Go generic**.

Choose to use one pharmacy so newly ordered medications are checked to be certain they won't interact badly with other meds you are taking. You can get to know the pharmacists as trained medical professionals; they can certainly be helpful to you.

Also, the pharmacist can tell you which over the counter (OTC) meds they recommend because not all are the same and might interact with your prescription meds. Be sure to ask about the safety of OTCs for you before taking meds for a cold.

You can also ask your pharmacist to get all your medicine on the same refill schedule. This will help you manage your medication refills more conveniently. Further, your long-term prescriptions can be filled for 90 days for further convenience.

Follow instructions for taking meds carefully because they are there for a reason. Meds that are to be taken with food may irritate the lining of an empty stomach. Avoid grapefruit juice with meds and taking calcium (milk, etc.) with antibiotics.

Take statins at bedtime, advises the British Heart Foundation. Here's why: Cholesterol production in the liver is highest after midnight and lowest during the morning and early afternoon, so statins are most effective when taken just before bedtime. New research suggests that the best time for people with hypertension to take their blood pressure pills is at bedtime rather than in the morning.

Antidepressants called selective serotonin reuptake inhibitors, or SSRIs, are taken in the morning because they can interfere with sleep, especially as you begin taking them, an expert says. Heartburn meds (Protein Pump Inhibitors, PPIs) need to be taken on an empty stomach, 20 to 30 minutes before breakfast.

But if you have mainly evening or nighttime symptoms, ask your doctor about taking Omeprazole 20 to 30 minutes before dinner on an empty stomach, since none of the PPIs truly lasts 24 hours.

However, many meds last 24 hours, which can reduce missed doses; plus, one might arrange to take all one's meds simultaneously.

Are You Supplementing Big Drug Companies by Tossing Good Meds?

Everything unfortunately expires, including drugs, both prescription drugs and OTC meds (over the counter meds). A 1979 law required all pharmaceutical and OTC producers to label their products with a date they would guarantee potency. Guess what? Their incentive is to sell you medicine, so? Sounds like the proverbial fox guarding the henhouse. **Scoundrels!**

Our military stockpiles a large amount of medicine in case it rapidly becomes needed and over time they became concerned about the cost of expiration dates. They commissioned a study by the FDA to determine how long meds actually lasted. The study showed almost all meds were just as good as when manufactured after 15 years!

Another well done report examined potencies of over 3,000 lots of 122 medications to see if different time of manufacture made a difference. They found that the average time beyond the expiration dates before any drop in potency could be detected was over 5 and 1/2 years.

Much more impressive, a researcher found 14 meds that were expired 28 to 40 years in a retail pharmacy in original, unopened containers. When these meds were tested for potency, strength was maintained to at least 90% levels of the original prescription.

There is a general consensus among experts that storing meds in the refrigerator further extends usefulness. There are a few exceptions: nitroglycerin, insulin, and liquid meds. Tetracycline, the antibiotic, questionably becomes toxic. However, the tetracycline toxicity was from a discontinued preparation and no other reports of harm from taking outdated drugs are available.

Have we all been throwing away perfectly good meds because we are being fed lies? No, because we are not informed, which is what we need to make correct choices.

An additional consideration that I have is taking medicine newly on the market on a long-term basis. In Canada, about one-fourth of newly released medications are recalled because of side effects. If a medicine has been on the market for years, I am reassured that long-term use is safe, which is another benefit of generics. They have been available for at least 20 years, which is the length of a patent's protection on the original script.

Getting the Most Out of Your Meds

The pharmaceutical companies have a great system of direct marketing to physicians. They send out drug reps in fewer numbers than in the past but they are still around going directly to the medical offices and clinics to convince the doctors that their company's product is better. Pharmaceutical companies are business companies; they promote more expensive medicines. They often come bearing gifts to medical prescribers.

The prescribers (physicians, nurse practitioners, and physicians' assistants) can be misled into costing their patients more with limited added benefit. Ask your prescriber whether there is a generic that will be as good. The medical profession is generally very professional but there are a number of bumps in the road in the corporate sections.

Another pharmaceutical marketing tactic is direct to patient advertising. TV ads are replete with smiling happy people because of buying expensive meds. Remember the past cigarette ads? If you get interested in asking your doctor for the advertised medicine, do it in the manner of asking for an opinion as whether the medicine will be worth a premium. There are studies showing that patients asking for a specific medicine or test often get it.

Medication's patent protection lasts 17 years, and then companies other than the developer can apply to produce competitive products, termed generic medications. Generic means without a trade name; generic is the chemical name of the medication.

Generic drugs cost 20% or even less than brand named ones because they don't share the cost of development. Are generic users settling for less quality? No, not at all. The FDA has stringent criteria for approval of generic medications. The chemical composition of active ingredients must be identical, and the absorption of the drug must be the same. This means the drug works the same way and is in the same amount.

Over 2,000 generic's absorptions were compared to the original brands and the generics averaged 96.5%, which provides the same clinical results as the brand name. Further, in dozens of medical studies, outcomes were compared and in every case study were identical.

The FDA monitors both classes of medications for adverse events the same to insure continued quality. Most non-generic drugs have alternatives in the same class, which will suffice. There are diabetes meds that have no generics to do what they do.

A possible difference is that generics may have different additives, other than the active ingredients, than the brand names, which can upset a few patients. Overall, there are few if any reasons for paying premiums for the same drug.

Another area of possible savings is in getting a prescription for an over-the-counter medicine if you take it on a regular basis. A person taking heartburn med Prilosec at 40 milligram daily pays considerably more than a $5 prescription of the same active ingredient. There is a yearly savings of $345 by prescription. If you require higher doses of non-narcotics pain relievers such as Aleve or Advil, there are modest savings with prescriptions. Get informed and be involved.

Tablet splitting can cut your cost for medications in half, but several steps are necessary to ensure safety. Some time-release medicines and capsules are not eligible for splitting. Tablets that are FDA approved for splitting will say so in the package insert and will be scored. Some tablets may be split that are not FDA approved, ask your health-care professional.

Use a pill splitter and do not split the entire bottle because split tablets can deteriorate over time. Do not split tablets that disintegrate; you can't be sure of the dosage.

Generally, larger quantities of the same medicines are cheaper. The standard amount is monthly but medicines taken long-term can be purchased for 90 days and be cheaper. And it saves the extra trouble of remembering refills and extra trips for pickup. Simplify, simplify, and simplify for a better life.

There are often many ways to do things, even taking your meds. But there is always a best way and a little knowledge about your medicines can be of considerable benefit in discovering the best way. I have always believed, as Gertrude Stein quipped, 'To be a difference, it has to make a difference.' So, what follows either is proven to make a difference or common sense from available facts make a difference very likely.

Improving Your Personal Medical Care

'Unfortunately, there's a slight disconnect between what's taught to doctors and what we know from chronotherapy research [when to take meds],' says circadian biologist Dr. Georgios Paschos of the University of Pennsylvania School of Medicine. 'Except for a few conditions, clinical medicine hasn't yet caught up with our findings.'

Nevertheless, he predicts, this will change in the next decade or two. I propose to catch you up right now in this chapter concerning the best way to reorganize your medical treatments.

What Dr. Paschos laments is that research investigating how to provide better medical results by timing medications is known but has not found its way into clinical medical practice.

Delayed clinical application is not a new drawback; medicine divides into two camps: physicians (MDs) who concentrate on providing and researching patient care and "basic scientists" (mainly PhDs) who concentrate on researching how our bodies work, how disease disrupts, and how medicine works to correct disease.

Having both degrees (MD, PhD) and experience in both disciplines, I appreciate how both work and that their professional communications are primarily group-based. A while back, an attempt to bridge the information gap foraged for a season; it promoted basic science more rapidly being put into practice and was termed translational medicine.

Nevertheless, we see medical communication still has gaps. This paper will inform the reader what is of importance that failed to make the break concerning medication usage.

Medicines can be taken by mouth (swallowed or held under the tongue), inhaled, injected with a hypodermic needle, or, gasp, (mostly in children) by rectal suppository. Obviously, injections are the fastest to work followed closely by inhaled or under the tongue methods.

One-third of adults experience some difficulty when swallowing solid meds. Obviously, moving the meds to the very back of the tongue and dispatching them with a large gulp of liquid helps. A study on the best way to swallow meds showed there is relief in extending the neck forward during swallowing or sucking bottled water from its bottle when swallowing solid meds.

Swallowed meds, however, depend on the particular medication's absorption curve. Since most medicine's beneficial actions depend on having a proper amount in the bloodstream (therapeutic range), knowing about the time it takes to reach beneficial levels and how long beneficial levels last is important and we will spend time on that aspect.

In general, meds that need to be taken infrequently are absorbed more slowly and are therefore eliminated more slowly.

Avoiding Adverse Drug Reactions

Meds always have drawbacks, termed side effects, or if severe enough, adverse drug reactions. Adverse drug reactions are by definition severe enough to require a trip to receive medical care. Side effects are results that are different than the medicine is designed to produce. They usually are mild with one exception—allergic reactions.

Allergic reactions range from itchy rashes to having the face swell to difficulty breathing. Having difficulty breathing is the most dangerous, swelling of the face or difficulty-breathing rates an immediate 911 call.

Adverse drug reactions are more common in elderly patients. In medical lingo, elderly means the transition between middle age and old (i.e., over 65 years). In medicine, old age then begins at 80 years. **Oh no!** Adverse reactions serious enough to be reported in Italy were 1.2% annually in persons over 65 years.

Unreported reactions are likely many times higher. In one large study, almost 7% of elderly hospital admissions were to treat adverse drug reactions.

Drugs have many side effects; look at the warning sheets included with your prescription. **Wow!** Those materials are not too helpful because they include many possibilities that are unlikely but included because of legal implications. Get information from your doctor. When a new medicine is prescribed ask, 'What should I look out for that would indicate side effects?'

The best information, however, is from the pharmacist for what reactions new meds might have.

A few drugs are inherently dangerous, such as blood thinners, chemotherapy meds, and meds to keep the heartbeat regular. Patients on dangerous drugs should follow instructions carefully and learn all they can about the medicine from their doctor and reliable sites on the internet.

Reliable sources are the Agency for Healthcare Research and Quality (www.ahrq.gov/.../btpills.htm), WebMD, and websites of academic institutions, such as Mayo Clinic and Johns Hopkins.

The most common serious adverse reactions are from drug interactions. The elderly often take a number of medicines because of multiple co-morbidities. One study had the average number of meds for 70 year olds at eight. The greater the number of meds taken the greater the chance of interactions.

Having a too large number of meds is termed polypharmacy and a movement is underway to reduce the number of meds in the elderly with polypharmacy. At least on your yearly checkup visit, you should review your meds with the doctor to make sure you need each one. On a cautionary note, discontinuing meds sometimes needs to be done gradually.

As the number of prescribing physicians increased, so does adverse drug reactions. Each additional prescriber increased the chance of adverse effects by almost a third. The problem is a lack of effective communication between prescribers. You, the patient, need to monitor medication changes.

The first line of defense is to inform your primary care doctor's office, probably through the doctor's assistant, that a new medicine is being added. Next, you need to check for drug interactions. Yes, your doctor should have examined your drug list and the pharmacy is supposed to do that, but you should always play it safe. Several websites have interaction checkers, which work well: WebMD and Walgreens are two.

Making Your Medical Care More Acceptable

Years ago, I was boarding a plane to lecture at a medical conference when my cell phone rang. It was Mom who wanted me to know she loved me because she was about to die. This was highly irregular because Mom was one of the most stoic people I knew. I immediately drove 200 miles to Tulsa and found Mom was correct; she had a pulse rate in the thirties and was about to die from heart failure.

She was overmedicated inappropriately with two similar heart meds, which had slowed her pulse rate to disastrous levels. I stopped her meds and by late afternoon, she was feeling much better. I took her to the best restaurant in Tulsa for dinner. I called her doctor, informed him of the overmedication, and requested that I be informed of future medication changes. Mom kept seeing him because he was so nice.

Judge your doctor by professionalism and results. The doctor should be aware of what you are taking just as you should. I fired a financial advisor because he did not know what my portfolio contained during our conversations. How can advisors advise without knowing particulars? Review your meds in detail with your doctor when new meds are added, or otherwise at least yearly.

Make no mistake: You are responsible for monitoring your meds. Bring a list of all of your medicines to each doctor visit. Include any supplements you are taking, so the doctor will be accurately aware of your therapeutic routine. Acts showing you take your therapy seriously will make your doctor more attentive.

I almost failed auto shop class in high school but whenever I was told I need auto repairs before wealthy enough to buy a new car, I would ask for explanations of why this needed to be fixed and more often than not, a cheaper alternative was offered.

During emergencies, knowledge of medications taken is important. Keeping a list of medicines for you and spouse in your wallet or on your smartphone is a safeguard to solve the problem if needed and have your wife do the same.

Medication errors are more common than patients realize. A few years ago, when I was prescribed a rare drug, a middle practitioner wrote for a dose that would have soon become an overdose problem. When I pointed it out, she was very embarrassed. The pharmacist would have almost certainly caught the glaring mistake, but the point is we must remain on guard. Had I not been a physician, I would not have known the dose was wrong.

To guard against errors, patients should know the major side effects of new medications, which is the second layer of protection because overdosing would be likely to have side effects. The list of side effects is usually included in an insert with prescriptions, read it.

Patients have responsibilities at the pharmacy as well. Make sure that the name on the medicine vial is yours. Most of the time, the pharmacist will meet with you before you get new meds, if not, ask to meet with the pharmacist. They should be good at telling you what the medicine is for what it does and what side effects it has. Pharmacists are trained specifically about medicines and their nuances.

As previously mentioned, when to take meds is rarely included with prescriptions. The drug labels tell you how many times a day to swallow them and occasionally advise you to take some with meals. However, our bodies have clocks that synchronize with sleep/wakefulness cycles.

For instance, statins that lower our cholesterol work by inhibiting the liver from making it. Our livers make the most cholesterol as we sleep, therefore statins are most effective when taken at bedtime. **Effective is important!**

Next, especially with once-a-day meds, there is a drug concept that is important—drug absorption curve. Aspirin is coated with a retardant to keep it from dissolving in the stomach and causing erosions. Such are labeled enteric-coated or safety-coated. Enteric-coated low-dose tablets are the recommended aspirins to take for wellbeing.

Their major function is to prevent heart attacks, among other benefits, by partly disrupting the clotting mechanism. The optimal time to achieve the highest level of aspirin in the morning is to take aspirin at night. Taking coated aspirin at night makes sense because the greatest numbers of heart attacks and the most serious ones occur in the morning hours.

People having arthritis pain should note when they have the worst episodes and time their NSAIDS pain meds four to six hours before. Usually, this means the arthritis meds should be started in the mornings before becoming active.

Medicines that are taken once a day and provide continued serum levels are termed extended release (ER). Many meds are available in ER form. Usually, that is the more desirable form because their absorption and reduction is slower that meds that must be taken more often. As a group, they should be taken at night because metabolism and a lot of risks slow as we sleep.

Non-compliance is common in the elderly. One can forget to take meds or forget they have taken meds. A Pill Organizer will help prevent this. Develop a routine to ensure compliance. Just before going to turning off the lights and going to bed, I need to do three things: set up coffee, get nightly water poured, and take meds. Establish a routine to take meds and stick to it. Pair it with other repetitive tasks so each reinforces the other.

There are meds that should be taken with meals and others that should be taken on an empty stomach. It does not always hold true, but a rule often applies that if the medication should be taken with meals, the pharmacist will place a label advising so on the prescription. If no label is present, take the medicine on an empty stomach, unless it upsets your stomach.

Pain meds are rarely labeled because they usually are taken as needed, but some meds, especially narcotics, should be taken with food to avoid an upset stomach.

There are some foods that should be avoided when taking certain medicines. When taking blood thinners, one should memorize that considerable list of potentially harmful foods and supplements. Grapefruit interacts with a number of meds. Particularly, grapefruit affects the absorption of cholesterol-lowering meds and some heart meds and may raise their levels in the blood dangerously high.

If you are taking those meds, it would be wise to substitute other citrus and avoid grapefruit altogether.

The liver and kidneys eliminate medications; medications don't just disappear. People with diseases of these organs likely will need to have doses reduced. When getting new prescriptions, patients with decreased function of these organs should remind the prescriber by saying, 'Does this dosage take my kidney problems into account?'

Making your medical care more acceptable: This is a yearly savings of $345. If you are requiring higher doses of non-narcotics pain relievers such as Aleve or Advil, there are modest savings with prescriptions. Get informed and be involved.

An additional consideration that I have is taking medicine newly on the market on a long-term basis. In Canada, about one-fourth of newly released medications are recalled because of side effects. If a medicine has been on the market for years, I am reassured that long-term use is safe, which is another benefit of generics. They have been available for at least 17 years, which is the length of a patent's protection.

I have always believed that when others embraced the premise that working harder or longer would bring success was true but the real secret to success was working smarter. The same applies to your health choices. **Absolutely!**

Wisdom is Ideal When Driving Your Automobile

Wisdom simply tells you what to do or not do next when given a certain situation. There is no undertaking (poor word choice) where wisdom should so constantly be applied than when driving your auto. Let's explore some auto driving wisdom.

Texas rates near the top among states in fatal accidents (fourth) from improper lane changes! It is common to see sudden unsignaled lane changes or a nut-job riskily changing multiple lanes at once, especially in heavily populated areas. If you are about to miss an exit, just go to the next one! **Don't be a nut-job!**

Be particularly careful about riding beside another auto for prolonged periods, especially if the driver appears distracted by devices or is weaving even slightly. It is not only a few dents incurred but slammed vehicles usually lose control and alongside our highways large immovable objects reside.

According to the Texas DPS law, as in many other states, one should signal for 100 feet before making a turn. In a few other states, the law is 200 feet. Personally, I use 200 feet as my minimum. I want the added safety of alerting others what I am about to do. Ensure safety for the times you have blind spots. I recommend signaling whenever a turn is to be made, even from a stop. There might be a pedestrian or bicyclist that you cannot see but wish to avoid. Allow them to avoid you.

My son was recently involved in a major accident which destroyed his auto by a driver who ran a red traffic light. Fortunately, thank Providence, he was not seriously injured. About two decades ago, at the Texas Medical Center, I had the same situation occur. A careless driver ran a red light, I went on green, and the wreck totaled my car. He hit my car's front and not my door or it would have been no more me.

So, here is the take home message: Since that accident, I have hesitated for a second or two when the traffic light turns green and looked both ways before stepping on the gas. I have seen other cars that were "rushing the red" pass safely on their way and then and only then, I did too.

According to a study by Owsley, 'the driving task is primarily visual in nature, and impaired vision is associated with increased driver discomfort, difficulty, and crash risk.' This especially was a factor when visual field reduction existed. Keep up to date on having your eyesight checked, yearly.

To emphasize the point: night driving is particularly hazardous; fatalities per mile driven are several times that of miles driven with the advantage of daylight. Also, according to government data, drunk driving as might be expected is much more common, especially from midnight to 3 am and weekends. Don't drive at night if your night vision is suboptimal.

The Necessary Decisions to Prevent Vehicle Collisions

Motor vehicle accidents are an enormous problem. Last year, according to the CDC, over 32,000 drivers were killed and over 2 million were injured. 712 traffic-related serious injuries result every day. The US has double the number of traffic deaths as do other developed countries. The Houston area is among the deadliest of the metropolitan areas.

Although, Texas ranks in the middle of states with 9.1 deaths per 100,000 population, the deadliest is Wyoming with 20 deaths per 100,000. Wild west!

Denial and complacency feed the factors we will discuss below. Operating a moving vehicle among other moving vehicles operated by other fallible human beings is inherently dangerous! We realize this as we are learning to drive, but we get complacent about the danger as we get more comfortable behind the wheel.

We are cognizant of the risks of certain behaviors, but because we have done them and nothing bad happened, we deny the danger and get comfortable doing them. Distracted driving is the number one cause of auto accidents. This includes texting, talking on the cellphone, and eating while driving. **Avoid.**

Next, the causes of accidents are speeding, drunk driving, reckless driving, rain, running red lights follow in that order.

About one-third of motor vehicle accidents with injuries are alcohol related. Not surprising, almost a third of serious motor vehicle accidents are associated with cellphone distractions as well. **Avoid those!** In simulator testing, driver's texting or talking on cellphones were found to have 3 to 4 times the risk of accidents. **Not a good idea**.

The damage from collisions of moving objects depends on the energy released by the collision. Moving objects possess kinetic energy: the size of the mass and its velocity. The formula is K.E. = ½ mass x the speed squared. If one doubles the mass of the vehicle and speed is constant, resulting damage doubles.

If speed doubles and mass remains constant, energy quadruples! This means the speed one is going rapidly increases the violence of a crash. The average car weighs 4,000 pounds, so a pickup truck weighing 8,000 pounds doubles the damage at similar speeds. Imagine now, the energy of a loaded eighteen-wheeler weighing 80,000 pounds! Collisions between passenger cars and trucks are not fair contests. **No way.**

To avoid crashes, we generally must apply brakes. The brakes turn the kinetic energy of our moving vehicle into heat. The faster we are going, the more energy there is to be changed into heat, and this takes time. Therefore, the faster we are going, the longer it will take us to stop, so our following distance must increase as our speed and/or vehicle mass increases.

Wet roads that reduce the coefficient of friction between the tire and road surface increase our stopping distance as well. A two second following distance is the base recommendation, with one second added for each factor that increases stopping distance, such as wet roads, heavier vehicle, pulling a trailer, etc.

Sensible Flashes to Steer Clear of Vehicle Crashes

Texas has the largest number of fatal accidents involving large trucks (>10,000 pounds) at 705 deaths in 2021. Drive defensively around large trucks because they have large blind spots, make wide turns, and cannot stop nearly as quickly as a car. Also, because of their weight (40 tons), their energy to damage a passenger vehicle will create 10 times that of another car.

I am careful about being around large trucks and spend as little time as possible alongside them.

Head on collisions are the deadliest. They compose only 2% of USA crashes but over 10% of auto crash deaths. The safest lane is the most right-sided lane if you are a careful driver with little chance to run off the road. Crashes off the highway can be deadly.

About 15% of fatal crashes in Texas involve large trucks; so be particularly alert when around them. Large trucks require up to 40% more space to stop so be careful not to allow them to tailgate your car. According to the American Association of State Highway and Transportation Officials, it takes alert drivers approximately 2 seconds to see a roadway hazard and react to it.

So, don't allow any vehicles to tailgate your car. Tailgating is a factor in one-third of accidents. Tailgating causes Phantom Traffic Jams. Have you ever been in stop and go tailgating traffic when there is no discernible reason? It seems to be a problem all the time in my highway driving.

How to get rid of them is to slow up until they get the idea and back off and simply pass you, or if they are incorrigible, use your emergency flashers that will confound most tailgaters! Highway Triumph though knowledge!

Just as in dog-human falls, there is a problem with deer-vehicle collisions. My daughter collided with a deer taking her son to school and totaled her car. The average cost of vehicle damage is about $4,000.

Wikipedia reports that there are 1,200,000 deer vehicle collisions a year in the US. Wow! I would have guessed 10,000. These collisions result in 200+ human deaths a year and I cannot find how many deer bite the dust. Glico recommends that in addition to slowing down in deer country that this should be done especially at dawn and dusk when they are most active.

Also, deer are most active in autumn months. If you see a deer, go very slow because they are pack animals and be especially careful when seeing a deer crossing sign. When on a multilane highway, the center lane is safest. Avoid swerving, brake instead, trees are more deadly to hit than are deer.

A long blast of you horn should scare them away from the road. Use bright lights when no cars are coming. Let's protect our horned friends, and ourselves too.

Rain (surprisingly) is more hazardous than snow. Sources do not say why but I suspect people are more careful when it snows. Do not speed on slickened roads as your car can plane out of control.

There Should Be Elation About Motivation Providing Salvation

To achieve and better yourself in this life you are given first requires motivation. Motivation is the mindset so that enough willpower is gathered to set about achieving a desired result. My mother repeatedly issued the challenge, from the time I could walk, that 'If you don't continually better yourself in this life you'll wind up as sorry as dirt,' and I most assuredly did not want that to happen. **Motivating!**

As Dolly Parton so aptly proclaimed, 'If you don't like the road you're walking, start paving another one.' And Mark Twain acknowledged, 'The secret of getting ahead is getting started.' When achieving any goal, getting started seems to be a stopping block for many of us and motivation is the method to make a start. At the gym I frequent, there is a sign stating "Believing you can do it and getting on is being half done".

Motivation is prompted by the perception of a need. Andrew Maslow proposed a hierarchy of human needs that are grouped by significance as Physiological (hunger, thirst), then Safety, then Social (love, friendship), then Self-esteem, and next Self-actualization (achievement of full potential).

Maslow postulated that the degree of fulfillment of these needs determined the degree of self-fulfillment. In other words, what is there in your life that you want utmost to enhance?

What aspect of your routine of living could be improved? No, more important, what aspect should be improved? When you reconsider your full potential, have you reached it? Most of us can always stretch our abilities just a bit, especially if we get into the habit of recurrently cultivating betterments in our lifestyles. **Think needs!**

In what aspect of your life have you settled into a drab let's just do as little as possible attitude? Before I retired and especially even before Covid, my mindset was to use time well to accomplish and most important avoid wasting time.

To be successful in achieving goals, correct methodology must be adhered to, and I obtained the right way often from the ideas of others. Consider a single feasible goal that can be divided into smaller tasks. Before starting, consider the benefits that will occur by achieving your goal. Bring family, friends, or better both for support into your confidence about your plans and seek their backing. Set reminders and times to complete each task.

The quality of our lives is reflected by our principles, values, and goals which are determinants of what we hold significant. **Come on quality**. My mother recurrently told me from the time I could talk, 'What determines how successful you are in life as a person is how many people you help.'

Naturally, we wish to make our lives and especially the lives of our loved ones better as we continue but how about others as well? I work to write about health matters to do so but there are nearly countless ways other's lives can be helped. There is no doubt that there is a great deal more personal gratification in our lives when we benefit others than when we benefit ourselves.

The Golden Rule provides the guidance that if we treat others as we would wish to be treated wholesome self-satisfaction is a gain that really happens and a feeling of living the good life is realized.

Life Is a Song and Dance If You Enhance Your Circumstance

Even the most cultured among us often do not know precisely what constitutes their reality. Often, we misguidedly consider it simply as a backdrop in which we survive. Your environment in the global sense includes your surroundings, all the people in direct contact, aggregate societal happenings, and how you think about these aspects.

Your reality is what you make it to be. **Evaluate and act**. Consider the total of your existence and how it enchantingly morphed into your present. Briefly detail the enhancements that added to your present-day province and then reflect on the impediments and how you overcame them. It will bring a smile and might make you feel like dancing. If so, go ahead, **dance!**

Place some humor in your life and your life will brighten up. After all, as the quote "Dance in the Rain" exuberantly instructs, life isn't about frightfully waiting for the storm to pass, it's about learning to dance in the rain. Dance!

As mentioned but notable, a very close Jewish friend experienced hard times yet always seemed to keep on top of it all. When things went south, he would vehemently shrug his shoulders and loudly say, 'this too will pass,' and go on with his life.

As my wonderful grandmother Nichols advised when troubles burdened, 'Just adjust your attitude.' I adjusted my bummer attitudes for the remainder of my life and improved outcomes considerably. Examine what has happened and particularly the why in detail. Carefully choose what you can and should do to deal with the state of affairs.

If you can do nothing to improve things, decide whether feeling remorseful will help, and if not, stop your internal torment and think of how to avoid similar problems in the future.

Terminate the run-through of habitually appreciating the good things in life most when they are gone. That nearly universal distortion cheats the perpetrator out of much satisfaction. Embellish your good fortune by fully appreciating the goods life has bestowed, especially family and good friends, repeatedly in the present moment. Make each moment count, and you will approach abundant life.

Stop and create a gratitude list in your mind, and appreciation will soar as your spirit rejoices. In doing so, think of three happenings in the last 24 hours that were refreshing. Make time to spend with your loved ones and friends, and when around them or communicating by phone, make them the sole purpose of your attention by avoiding distractions.

Be thankful for your plentiful meals because there are more hungry people in the world (over 825 million) than almost 2.5 times the population of the US. We are abundant in sustenance with huge grocery stores and nearly countless fast-food shops waiting for hungry people in the USA.

Express your affection by noticing the good things and delightfully complimenting others when deserved. Dispense appropriate hugs. Appreciate good friends willingly but especially let loved ones know you care. Make, heartfelt thank you, one of the most often spoken phrases out of your mouth. Make your life gratifying by knowing your most pleasurable activities and repeating them often.

The Emphasis of Emotional Intelligence Is Healthfulness

With the gargantuan destructive impact which the dreaded pandemics bring trends have developed to understand and improve lifestyle. It is appropriate to have appraised how to enhance contentment during extensive displeasure by improving one's lifestyle. A recent nascent attempt by scientific psychologists is through emotional intelligence. Embracing that enhancement of self-control can greatly enrich one's life.

Personal emotion is unlike many important aspects of living, it is considered to just transpire and it does so if no control is applied and like other aspects of our personality, it can always become better-quality. **Always choose self-control!**

According to the American Psychological Association, emotion has three components, an experience occurs in a person's mind which triggers one's bodily physiology to respond in smiles or scowls, and behavior is adjusted accordingly. **Wow!** The human mind is divisible into conscious selves and a much larger subconscious division.

This spontaneous instinctive brain tells our awake "self" what mood to accept and our conscious self behaves accordingly. Without intervention and taking control, our emotional steerage is on autopilot. **Our submarine selves!**

Emotional intelligence presumes that we may amend our emotions consciously to achieve a much better-quality value-added lifestyle. Do away with aftermaths that need to think "if I had only done it another way it would have worked out fine". It is a common bummer to rehash events that went south and stipulate the result would have been better if I had done thus instead of that. **Whoa, you didn't know!**

To cultivate the capability for possessing and then enhancing emotional intelligence, one must become aware of your momentary emotional state. Continually inquire as to "what am I feeling at this moment" and begin to notice when your emotional status modifies. Then ask yourself why is this happening and in what way can I receive the best in my life by managing my emotional state?

While sadness might be considered the most common powerful negative emotion, stress seems to be the leading disrupter.

Stress is a reaction our mind and body has from the consideration of something that needs to be done or will happen or has happened and generally stress can easily get out of control unless well-ordered properly. Tell yourself about the many times you have overcome similar difficulties and smile as you realize **this too will pass**.

Realize that you are in control of your life and be reassured you will overcome life's obstacles without beating yourself up. **Treat your "self" better!**

Promise your "self" that although we cannot control everything it often comes out better than we expect and don't waste effort worrying about things you can't control. Be a positive thinker concentrating on what is good in your life and choose to never overextend yourself emotionally.

The next steps are to consider and gage the emotional states of anyone with whom you have a relationship because using proper communication you can impart some of your emotional intelligence and enhance their lives. Expanding the concept, note the overall mood of any group you are with and stay in a healthy framework by keeping a positive mood toward eventual outcomes.

This seeking and securing will not happen at once but over time as you continue to analyze and improve your overall emotional intelligence becoming better able to dance life's tune amazingly well. **Just keep going.**

Taking the Self Off the Shelf, We Must Agree Helps to See the Real Me

This concept of self as a definable entity dates back a long time and its developers includes such notables as Rene Descartes and Sigmund Freud. It relies heavily on what our conscious brain concludes but self's processes are by and large subconscious.

The challenge of knowing about our innermost self initially may sound hackneyed or unintelligible generating a response of course I am my own self and I understand myself explicitly.

However, self is the conclusive core of one's being. Each of our selves differentiates from all others who are or have ever been and in doing so illuminating one's uniqueness, the self. We briefly brush the surface when we identify favorites, such as my favorite color, time of year or the many others.

The self is our being's foundation from which come our standards, needs, values, principles, and beliefs that create our personalities. Self is the compass that directs us and the framework to evaluate our environment, especially characterizing situations and gauging others around us. By knowing our personality's beliefs, we can hone our lives by coordinating our intuitive foundational person with our conscious activities.

Set aside a time when you will be undisturbed or distracted and get the contemplation underway. What are the happenings and individuals in your lifetime that have shaped your life cycle and your innermost self? Who and what made you who you are? This should be a deep examination of who you really are and refrain from embarking on a "what if something else had happened". What actually happened certainly come about.

What principles and values are most significant in guiding your life's choices? How have these beliefs motivated your lifestyle? Are you pleased with what you have accomplished? Make a mental list of major accomplishments. Most of us have a few down blips on a line that just kept on heading upward as time went by.

Keep returning to your inner self's voice that will point toward your special truth. Identify what could be enhanced in your self's repertoire and vow that your consideration can be implemented.

Consider what should be improved to establish a better milieu for you, loved ones, and associates. Seriously evaluating your inner-self likely will improve your personal emotional intelligence which is a substantial boost to your happiness and that of your loved ones. Guiding our lives through improvements in our behavior by adjusting our self can be a fantastic improvement.

Recognize that you are responsible for your happiness and that you can substantially impact the happiness of those around you. Ask yourself more often about feelings that happen and gradually have the "core self" achieve the perspective desired by your fully "mindful self".

Try to reduce your judgments of others based on previous incidents either good or bad, unless danger is involved. Those occurrences are judging an occurrence because it just looks the same as something earlier. In other words, unless danger is involved, delay judgement until specific circumstances occurs. Knowing more about crucial subjects is continually better and what is more important than your personal self?

Get Confident That Betterment of Contentment Is Triumphant

The quality of each of our lives is directly related to the quality of your thoughts and ideas. Too often we don't direct our thinking but if we adjust our emphasis the abundance of life has much more to offer. Correct!

Personal goals in life are important and should be sensibly thought out because attaining one's goals gives one's life purpose. Consequently, just what should our personal goals be? Frequently, they involve several themes including family, occupation, status, and affluence, but I would suggest that achieving contentment with your life should be right at the uppermost.

Contentment means to be satisfied or even pleased with what you yourself have done, your status in the world, and personal surroundings including things but mostly valuing people.

Contentment is important to relaxing one's lifestyle stress and brings about pleasurable conditions. **Find satisfaction**. It is important to rethink your surroundings and overall lifestyle periodically, especially in troubling times such as pandemics, and to realize that most of us in the USA have an abundance of necessities to live a good life and be comfortable.

If one has contentment, it does not mean giving up ambitions, instead it means focusing on the time at hand which is how you are presently living now and does not preclude having dreams for the future. It does not mean being troubled that your present is not adequate. There are personalities which constantly need to have more. **Don't be one!**

Decide if you have enough, which almost all of us have actually more than enough. We all should be seeking what for us is the ideal life. If you have enough to eat, comfortable surroundings with people you care about who care about you and have health sufficient to live a meaningful life then your present is sufficient, and you should recognize the adequacy in your personal present-day.

Accepting that your life is sufficient will allow you to receive contentment. **Get it!**

Don't predetermine when your contentment will happen such as basing your happiness on achieving certain goals and delaying it until the particular events happen. A good bit of our contentment becomes misplaced to our childhood learning experiences. When positive happenings occurred, our parents or our teachers would tell us to become pleased.

Those teaching us focused on external dealings. But this behavioral arrangement limits the internal self from sustaining a pattern of contentment with our lives that makes our "self" a happier mostly satisfied person. In other words, don't limit your satisfaction and internal rewards to future events which may not come about soon or at all. If you need to limit some considerations, limit negative thoughts.

Contentment tells your inner emotional determining self, 'You may and should be happy because your present-day situation is superb.' Also, avoid any and all what if considerations. Some of the saddest people I have ever met believed that life should be fair on their terms. I have been decent, and I don't know why this could have happened is a commonplace renouncement. Morality confers rewards and punishments but only in an offhand manner.

As an alternative, cultivate gratitude robustly concentrate on what you have. Almost all of us have habitable and safe surroundings. Enough nourishing food and loved ones and friends. **Come on in contentment**.

It is Prudential and Sometimes Essential to Maximize One's Chock-Full Potential

One of the truly vital words to keep in mind, especially when younger, is potential. The concept of potential is a challenge when it becomes how do I achieve my full potential? When young, it obviously is appropriate to have the need to be somebody noteworthy through developing grown-up skills. But let's each accept the challenge to repcatcdly cxamine and reach or even better our potential. **Yes!**

Optimistic potential is the true realism that one is capable of amassing the ability to make something highly desirable happen. It is a benchmark which challenges an individual to achieve a given goal generally of attainment.

One's personal potential must be conceived by each adult and in doing so, a "want me to be" mindset should be envisioned. Different potentials emerge as we go through life and school potential, becomes work potential, becomes career advancement potential, and becomes stages of retirement life potential. In the best framework, potential is a continuing journey with an ultimate goal of continuing to enhance one's lifestyle.

An illuminating interaction when I was with a group of smart professionals was to ask, 'If you were to choose a word to describe the difference between mediocrity and excellence, what would it be?' Many absolutely snappy retorts resulted. My best selection was anticipation. Stepping up to duties or challenges is best done when prepared by anticipating the situation, especially when health or safety is concerned.

Consequently, we should seek out our potential to anticipate a more rewarding future.

First, we need to determine what we would realistically like to attain and what needs to be undertaken for that to take place. Since tomorrows always continue to be alive throughout life, we need to repeatedly make the effort to place the realizing of potential as a mainstay on the way to being the best I can be. Do happen!

Substantial progress in one's standard of living can be assured if the Roman dictum articulated by Horace "carpe diem" is adhered to in one's life. This astonishing initiators' challenge literally translates as "pluck the day", which in modern times instructs us to "seize the day".

Horace's entire statement enthusiastically challenged to make the most of each day we are given and not delay while waiting for tomorrow because today done well will deliver us fabulous tomorrows. Further, one added key interpretation is that by seizing the day we should enjoy all the pleasures offered each day. Amen!

Applying the "constructing a building" metaphor, there are a number of necessary actions to be taken to achieve actualization of potential. As mentioned, the goal to be reached should be clearly defined and steps taken in proper order. Knowing one's full potential is essential but appropriate actions are absolutely necessary. Too often once the goal is apparent, and mostly it will be, we merely let it slide. Well, not any more for potential seekers.

Too often we focus on the past which we can only learn from but never change. Potential deals with the future and potential dwells in the future. Focus and energize there and your futures will shine brighter. Consider the marvelous satisfaction resulting from reaching full potential when you can genuinely exclaim, 'I have done all that is needed to do my best and be my best.' Amen!

You can Make Your Life Astute if You Troubleshoot Starting with a Reboot

The ultimate key to living the finest life one is capable of is to perfect the way it is lived by polishing your self's lifestyle. Lifestyle is gradually implemented by your family, educational level, moral training, romantic experiences, and the many additional encounters molding the inner self's beliefs.

- The most unbelievably complex part of a human body in one's living biosphere unquestionably is the conscious brain and its counterpart one's subconscious mind in the nonliving world is a modest but similarly intricate supercomputer, both entities use energy to function collecting information and amazingly assembling huge volumes of content to arrive at conclusions. **Wow, two brains!**

When the computer glitches happen, a simple but magnanimous procedure termed **reboot** generally renovates functioning back to normal. This simple on-off switch seemingly magically resets otherwise jammed malfunctioning programs to routine and the rebooted computer achieves normal status. Glitches happen because over time there is an accumulation of unneeded scripts causing hiccups which are removed by rebooting.

This column has focused for some time on reengineering everyday life so that we can be the best we can be. Even when we feel like shouting, 'This is as good as it gets,' the mood will not last long, but reengineering can make it happen more often. **Let good times roll!**

To initiate a reboot, isolate and be mindful only of your self, not of the non-self-environment from the outside world. Our selves have all the complex methods and routines propelling us to function as individuals leading independent lives in a vast complex world. But we need to come up to the realization whatever plans we have for reaching our goals maximally need to be properly adhered to rather than just given passing attention. **Give attention where needed!**

Meaningful personal rebooting allows focusing on eradicating shoddy segments of our persona which includes remorse, guilt, distaste of others, and especially, fear that something unpleasant is looming.

Look to such instances in your past which you regret and realize that keeping detrimental considerations from the past is like not taking out household garbage. It confers no value and only begins to stink up your lifecycle.

Life generally accumulates baggage because our cave-dweller brain focuses on serious incidents to stay alive. Rebooting dictates to decide that the past is past and has no place in the now. Expect the rebooting to remove your unwanted baggage and produce a clean slate for your mental being. Then you can restart and replace old habits with new more exuberant lifestyle and get "aha"! moments.

I must caution that I am not trained in psychiatry. However, I remember that I made one of the highest grades in psychiatry in medical school, enough so the chairman called me in and asked if I was going into psychiatry, but I replied no because I would just sit and analyze myself. The professor was not amused. **Aha!**

What Are the Grassroots Attributes of Fruits and Veggies?

There is no vagueness about the certainty of health benefits from ingesting fruits and vegetables or that the quantity consumed is directly related to the value received. Consumption of fruits and vegetables contribute to one's health span which contributes to lifespan. Start with inferior building material and you get inferior results. What we eat is used by our cells to repair and maintain our bodies.

For **goodness sake,** don't use inferior material. You wouldn't do so in building your home. Also, living cells function and exist because of our biological furnaces producing life-giving energy.

We have been and continue to be bombarded with guidance to eat more fruits and veggies but just as everything in life, fruits, and veggies vary or they would not have different monikers. The important variation is in their nutritional value to our bodies. **Yes!** I declare these facts because I do not wish to appear overly punctilious. If one goes to a racetrack to bet on winners, it is important to know the favorites. **Yes!**

In research studies evaluating multiple veggies and fruits, the nutritional value of top-raters can be four or five times the underdogs and popularity does not necessarily match nutritional value. OMG!

Here's a list of 5 healthiest fruits that you should include in your daily diet: Berries. Be it blackberries, cranberries, strawberries or blueberries, berries of all kinds are super nutritious. Apple is one super-fruit that can prove to be quite beneficial in your weight loss passage. Also, include watermelon and oranges.

Fruits you should avoid if you are trying to lose weight include the following: Any high-calorie fruit should be consumed less often to lose weight including avocados and grapes. While they are great for overall health, grapes are loaded with sugar and fats, which makes them the wrong fruit to eat while on a strict weight loss diet.

Dry fruits are relatively high in caloric content by weight because of the absence of water. Avoid them to lower calories and lose weight.

The healthiest vegetables on Earth include spinach. This leafy green tops the chart as one of the healthiest vegetables in a number of reliable studies. Next, closely behind are carrots, broccoli, garlic, brussel sprouts, kale, green peas, and Swiss chard.

Dietary modifications to include more fruits and veggies lower the rate of the diseases which are the most likely to put us away. One well designed study last year further estimated that those who ate the recommended amounts of fruits and veggies reduced their cancer risk by 40%! Also, the risks of stroke and other devastating happenings are reduced by dietary changes from red meat and other animal proteins to fruits and vegetables. **Yes!**

Further, and to sum up, the CDC scientists have cautioned repeatedly that only 10% of Americans eat the recommended quantity of fruits (1 and 1/2 to 2 cups) and veggies (2 cups or 2 and 1/2 cups) daily. **Let's do better!**

Slowing Aging to Keep
It from Raging

Aging can be considered to have a number of different phases. We generally think about the process of advancing through life in term of changes in physical appearance and behaviors. Signs that indicate the stage include childhood's phases, followed by adolescence, adulthood, and then finally grey hair, a few wrinkles, and hopefully some wisdom. Whereas, a biologist can look at cells under a microscope and see changes that announce the AGE OF CELLS—WHERE AGING ACTUALLY HAPPENS. But, with no buts about it, all life and the process of our aging is profoundly molecular.

As everyone knows, wrinkles appear prominent in areas exposed to the sun. Exposure is fun but produces aging molecules called oxidants which reduce the amount of collagen (the filler beneath the skin) resulting in sagging and reduces elastin that works like stretch material to give the skin a "good fit". Hair is produced by hair follicles that enclose the fastest growing cells in the body. The hair color is from pigment cells which produce melanin; they age fast or slow depending on the body's concentration of aging molecules.

These details are declared to ding-dong your attention and hopefully get you to buy into the idea that you want fewer aging molecules and more antiaging ones—fur sure. Molecules in our living bodies do specific tasks because of their complex molecular structures; change their structure and they stop doing their jobs. The cells are damaged thereby and they age. The extent of aging depends directly on the amount of aging molecules in your body.

Our bodies produce energy for life in crinkly tiny cellular ovens. The energy comes from well-controlled chemical "fires" that produce aging molecules as a byproduct. Think of the aging molecules as sparks from an actual fire because like sparks they can be harmless or damaging depending on whether they land on and damage essential molecules. Aging molecules are termed Free Radicals because they are relentlessly searching for a body's molecule which they can attach to and change. Over time damage accumulates at a rate depending on the rate of the radical's production. Consuming large amounts of calories, especially sugar, floors the metabolic GAS PETAL.

The remedy is to increase the number of antiaging molecules in your body. These miniscule "fire extinguishers" that shield you are termed antioxidants because they neutralize the aging molecules like a catcher's mitt traps a baseball. YEA! These little antiaging darlins' have two sources; they are made by the body and are contained in what we consume.

Every molecular process that is potentially harmful has a countermeasure to limit damage. Increased energy production from physical activity sensitizes antiaging processes. If you want your body to be antiaging focused Get More Active.

Other living creatures have the same antiaging setups as we do, especially plants. When we consume them, we can absorb their antiaging molecules and benefit depending on the amounts present. Berries, beans, tree-derived nuts, green leafy vegetables, and dark chocolate are super-duper antiaging indulgences. Consume Wholeheartedly.

Keeping Our Caveman Mentation Under Control

Studies have shown that a segment of our thinking influencing our behaviors is genetic and just happens. It brings forth the question of who gave us our foundational behavioral genes. Our genetic makeup constituting Homo Sapiens, or in Latin "wise man", appeared as long as 300,000 years ago as cave dwellers ruled the earth.

These early prototypes secured dominance in the living creature world among larger and fiercer beasts because of an upright two-legged stance freeing the arms and so called prehensile or grasping hands.

Using those two attributes, they could throw objects to injure other creatures while at safe distances, but single caveman warriors would have remained no match for saber-toothed tigers. But a hunting party with many warriors throwing weighty objects would indeed be deadly. Thus, to survive, cave people must belong to a tribe.

These tribe-belonging survivors that lived and bred past on their genes to us which is part and parcel of our being rooted in group mentality. Group mentality foremost means that we consider groups as our identities; this includes one's country, state, city, schools, clubs, and places of worship among other categories. We identify by being fans of our various groups.

"Group think" should be considered but must not be followed without careful personal consideration. Carefully consider each circumstance as to whether it is right for you to go along with the group.

Our ancient ancestors were opportunistic eaters, mainly when hunters found prey and it is obvious that those who ate more food when available were survivors.

Prehistoric survival was calorie based and fat has twice as many calories than other foods and since sugar is utilized directly, it gives an immediate vitality boost enough of both would be highly desirable if rapid actions were required to survive. Eat all you can to store up energy became the ancient's mantra. Being a desirable glutton made one a happy survivor.

Presently, we have abundant food and no need of overeating to survive. Therefore, we need to suppress those caveman urges that cause obesity. The more primitive thinking keenly wants to feel good because there were so much stressful happenings. The ancients remembered what made them feel better and repeatedly did the limited feel better activities available to them.

Now when stressed, we automatically desire do something satisfying to feel better. We may binge eat, drink alcohol, or take drugs as pick-me-ups. **Wrong.** Resolve problems that arise by rationally appraising what has happened. Realize that disappointments you have endured have all resolved and punishing yourself is not a solution, it only made you feel worse.

Remember the veracity the philosopher Nietzsche proclaimed, 'Whatever does not kill you makes you stronger.'

If the problem will resolve itself by next week, it is irrelevant. Sensibly appraise the problem unemotionally because emotion clouds reality and flares difficulties emphasizing troubles which rational persons do not need. The positive nature of circumstances is almost always within reach.

When my new car was damaged by a stoplight runner, I was relieved that no one had been injured and the responsible person had the means to fix my car. **Yes!**

Decree to Foresee a Carefree Reality and Have a Jamboree

In our surrounding material world, which backdrops our reality of existence, everything that happens has a cause. Otherwise, it is magic, and magic is just an entertaining illusion and illusions are only make-believe. Importantly, our realities are composed of portions that are participatory and portions that we are uninvolved.

Our immersive relationship with reality which is the collective of all activities we participate in and from which our awareness patterns and similarities come about. We alter this marvelous reality better if we embrace a successful lifestyle.

Dr. William Glasser, a gifted psychiatrist, created a remarkably brilliant method to examine and adjust one's personal reality for a more gratifying lifestyle. His method is termed Reality Therapy because it coaches readjusting decisions and actions for a more splendid daily life. Our emotional tiffs occur because our performance drops beneath our expectations.

My mother repeatedly issued the challenge, as far back as kindergarten, when I achieved something even if excellent such as getting an A on tests, 'Don't you truly believe that you could have done better. Now tell me what you will do next time to improve?' **Yes, improve!**

Above all, we are in control of our lives. Even when others are in authority, your choice to obey or not is still paramount. Therefore, we each bear the responsibility for actions determining most of our reality's happenings. Reality Theory emphasizes that optimizing behaviors from choices that satisfy our needs is paramount to a pleasing lifestyle. **Satisfy self!**

Normally, when considering our personal needs, we consider the essential needs of food, shelter, transportation, education, health, and a few others for survival.

The most authoritative needs list I have come across, and is generally considered to be finest, is from a psychologist named Maslow. He hits the nail on the head as already mentioned with survival essentials and then aspects of how one feels about one's self.

Those needs are physiological needs, safety needs, love and belonging needs, esteem needs, and self-actualization needs. Design and institute lifestyles to meet your needs.

Never Forget Your Biggest Asset Is a Well-Structured Mindset

Nurturing one's purpose in life is highly commendable because, as pithily revealed in medical literature, it results in a more contented, fulfilled, healthier, and a longer life. Desirable indeed! An objective in bettering personal purpose is to enhance your Mindset. Mindset is the self's fixed beliefs about life and lifestyle which guides decision making resulting in choices directing behaviors. Mindset is who you really are innermost.

Thus, our mindsets are the foundations of our very being and lifestyles. Just as strong foundations of our houses assure stability and endurance, personal enhanced wellbeing has the same benefits. The Bible metaphorically declares that one's personal foundational mindset when weak as when built on sand will not withstand the rigors of life but will heartily endure when built on solid rock. (Matthew 7:26)

In the broadest categorization, mindset may be dubbed positive or negative. A positive approach is a strong "just do it" versus "I am faced with difficulties I cannot deal with". Alan Rufus, a gifted life coach, put the notion succinctly as 'Life is like a sandwich, birth as one slice, and death as the other. What you put in-between your slices is up to you. Is your sandwich tasty or sour?' Developing a positive mindset is similar to securing a sous-chef to make your sandwich full of flavor. **Indeed!**

A good start is to reinforce and fully support your mindset's gratitude forte. Gratitude is the subject matter and contributes significantly to life satisfaction and general health in the medical literature with over 2,000 medical science papers on the subject. Gratitude ushers in satisfaction and is supremely positive.

From gratitude, gradually can come a more positive mindset conceivably becoming "yes, I can", which is the belief in self and promotes a healthy mindset. Being grateful for your abilities, accomplishments and surroundings encourages deep inner contentment. Belief in yourself and your abilities as your mindset strengthening allows you to expand boundaries set in the past and place brand new aspirations as goals.

Learn from the past and then let the past go. A forgive yourself mindset is a pathway to conviction that you are on the corridor life offers to reach high ranking goals and then achieving ever grander aspirations as you live. A substantive mindset will keep your actions on a higher much more productive pathway. Discard frustration it only serves to rob your ability to think through problems and suitably adapt.

Success in life needs belief in oneself. I was faced with many desperate situations in a long heart surgery practice and not once that I can remember did my team did not start with a belief that the situation would not be solved. **Solve the damn problem!**

Likewise, appreciate when you have succeeded for more mindset inspiration. After most desperate salvages, when completed, I would stand straight and loudly proclaim, 'Once again science, talent, and knowledge overcomes poverty, ignorance, and superstition.' **Yea!**

Routines for Reaching a Rewarding Lifestyle

Regular required happenings in life are without frustrations if habitual constructive routines are established. Especially true when individual habits add to one's contentment and health.

Such an event is when one goes to one's personal vehicle to go on an errand. I usually require three standard objects kept in separate places from my wardrobe, car keys, wallet, and sunglasses. These always reside in their designated spots. Also, additional objects such as a mask during epidemics cannot be forgotten if placed with the car keys.

With the dreaded Covid lurking, a mask by the keys is never forgotten. Another time when I ask if anything needs to be taken or left behind is when I go up eighteen stairs to my office. Yes.

A calendar app in my phone is routinely used to reinforce recollection of upcoming necessary events and my app has two alerts and I use them on the day before and the day of the event. In my office are calendars of 3 months where events are indicated and if important in red figures.

All of my loved ones birthdays, graduations, and other notable events are posted a week before the occurrences if it is planned to send a congratulatory card to be assured of arrival.

With age, we may experience waning memory which can be irritating to considerable extent. This occurs less in our visual memory than in other aspects such as auditory. An often encountered aspect is names of people or lists of items you need to purchase. Cement names by imagining the name on a paper held by the individual with their face clearly visible.

Remembering what needs to be done without fail can be accomplished by placing a calendar in an obvious, often visited site with such things as birthdays and other events to be planned are listed.

When leaving the house, routines apply to safeguard an enjoyable outing. A prophylactic trip to the restroom whether felt necessary or not avoids later possible inconveniences. Also, looking at weather forecasts on one's cellphone helps to make preparations such as when to take an umbrella.

Impeding the Indignity of Imbalance with Senior-Hood

Each year over 25 million older Americans suffer falls. This amounts to 1 out of every 3 people over 65 years of age. Every 13 seconds, an American has a serious fall and every 20 minutes someone who fell dies. Oh my! The risk swells to half of people after 75 years of age falling annually. Falls are the leading cause of trauma-related death and disability in America, by far.

Over 2.5 million ER visits are from falls and 700,000 of those who fell are admitted to the hospital. This results in over 30,000 deaths a year. OMG! Lightning strikes which seem more ominous, average 51 deaths a year.

The damage from a fall that resulted in a hospitalization was not completed on hospital discharge; 20% or 1 out of every 5 did not return to independent living. And the overall mortality rate within a year caused by falling was an additional 19%! Also, having taken a fall is a predictor of future falls.

The most common fall-prone area is the bathroom. Dangerous areas are wherever there are tile floors especially if they get wet. Place non-slip rugs there and night lights are necessary. Another distraction and fall causing mechanism is tripping over a dog. Among persons stating that their fall was dog related and almost half were serious enough to require hospitalizations. Almost all of those required operations. Apparently, trying not to hurt one's pet altered the faller's self-protection mode.

Protection from falls primarily involves two aspects: balance and leg muscle strength. People with balance difficulties have double the risk of falls. Numerous studies have proven that exercise programs improve balance. In the FAME Study, exercise at home reduced participant's falls by 54%. Also, those who fell had less serious injuries. Important medical studies tend to have names and thus should be considered more important.

In another study, people at risk for falls (balance problems or prior falls) were started on weekly balance exercises and their balance, muscle strength, reaction time, physical functioning, and general health status improved. And they had 40% fewer falls.

Another study (the Sunbeam Program) enrolled at risk adults living in 16 residential care facilities. They trained 2 hours a week, seeking prevention, and had 55% fewer falls than the control group and had no serious falls during follow-up. Pretty remarkable and darn, no, damn good insurance.

Lesser factors associated with falls are poor eyesight, inappropriate shoes (backless, smooth leather soles, and high heels), and household factors (clutter, poor lighting, and no railings on stairs). For a number of reasons have eye exams at 40 years of age and then on a regular basis according to your ophthalmologist's recommendation.

Medications that cause unsteadiness should be avoided in people who are unsteady with slow gaits and those who have had falls. Take a medicine list to your pharmacist.

More essential information on how to avoid major pitfalls in life can be found at drjimshealthtips.com. Furthermore, if you send your name and email address to me at jwjones@bcm.edu, I will include you in periodic health info that I run across.

What Does Commitment to Religious Beliefs Do for You Right Now?

Religion offers a prodigious prearrangement for a better afterlife to believers but does it offer benefits right now to individuals which exceeds the efforts spent practicing their religion? Securing a mansion in the afterlife is highly desirable but **how about right now?** In a very large study, over 20,000 subjects, life satisfaction, character strengths, and orientation to happiness were stronger in those who actively practiced a religion.

Furthermore, believing and having religious affiliations offered no benefit without practicing the religion actively.

Practicing a religion does not have to be limited to attending religious services. Daily private prayer has been shown to produce significant health benefits. Further, religious activity was shown to provide the most benefit if started before the onset of health problems.

Longevity is increased in those practicing religious activities but other confounding factors rather than the religion per se, such as support and additional socialization might be the reason. Musick explored alternatives and found a 30% reduction in mortality over a 7.5 year study. This was after elimination of the influence of possible confounding healthy behaviors!

Studies have confirmed that practitioners of religion live longer by avoiding death and more people die from heart attacks and stroke than any other causes. A study illuminated why: the markers (blood tests) for having future vascular problems were measured and were significantly lessened in religious people attending services. **Wow!**

The study participants (over 10,000) were tested and the positive criteria were attending religious services 40 or more times within the last year. Thus, it seems religious adherent's bodies biochemistry responded favorably.

Religious observance, termed religiosity, has many accompanying values. In a study of children's religiosity in high risk children who had family with serious disruptive problems, high risk children that were noted to be religious were 64% to 76% less likely (depending on the diagnosis) to experience psychological problems as they grew older. **Wow!**

However, discerning people desire to understand the "how did this happen"? Did God look down and favor these children? Perhaps, but since God, according to the holy literature and available experiences, seems to employ physical methods—not magic the individual benefits were from religiosity. Among all the psychological traits known to science, **resilience** has the most influence in reducing aging's detrimental outcomes.

Scientific studies looked at the degree of the influence spirituality had on resilience and it was considerable. **So, bounce back!**

In another study, older people who had religious doubts such as my illness is because "God abandoned me" were more apt to die. So, don't put any negative beliefs into your situation. **Please!**

A scientifically oriented mind might consider that deeply religious scientists might be biased toward religion's benefits. However, there are thousands of positive papers on various ways of examining the subject of the helpful personal effects that religion can bestow. Before each major operation, I asked patients to meet with a religious person their own or the hospital Chaplin, and I had the lowest mortality rates in the published literature!

Go to drjimshealthtips.com for the references. **Amen.**

Happiness: How Does One Grab It and Maximize It?

A number of things people consider important frequently are relegated to being just backdrops of life, including love and especially happiness. They will occur at the proper times because that is the way we are constructed. I recently had a good friend tell me, 'I have never been a happy person. That is just the way I am.'

Well, each of us determines the way we are. Some of the unhappiest people I ever met were those who believed life must be fair. Life works on a set of logical principles we define as physics, chemistry, economics, and many other categories, not what we believe is deserved. A popular song from twenty-five years ago was titled *Every Rose has its Thorn*. Yes!

The Prophet Matthew reiterated, 'Rain falls on the good and bad.' Ergo: do the best you can with the hand you are dealt.

Happiness is one of the greatest driving forces of human nature, barely behind self-preservation. It is right up there with "unalienable rights of life and liberty and the pursuit of happiness" in our Declaration of Independence. Thus, as we all know, we have a right to pursue happiness so it is important that we know how.

Happiness is a mental status that is created from an emotion generated from living a good life. So, happiness is secondary to other things that we do to promote a "good life".

The famous German philosopher Hegel best defined true happiness as a reward you give yourself from attaining a desire. Most of our efforts are aimed at producing happiness when our goals are reached. We want to be liked, productive, successful, and many other positive goals and so we go to great lengths to achieve those results.

Three aspects of subjective wellbeing can be distinguished: evaluative wellbeing (or life satisfaction), hedonic wellbeing (transient feelings of happiness, pleasure), and eudemonic wellbeing (sense of purpose and meaning in life). In essence, the three represent evaluations of past, present, and future statuses.

We surely can find happiness where it resides, in the positive quality of our thoughts about people and events. Remember that every cloud even rainclouds have silver linings. Look for the silver linings.

My personal take away observation for the happiness bank is when I have considered the future, nothing I have thought would turn out bad, turned out as bad as I considered it might be. And most everything I considered would be good, turned out to be better than I thought. Look for the silver linings. **They abound!**

Pedometers were used to measure physical activity in older adults and their measured physical activity correlated with their satisfaction with life. The Netherlands Twin

Study has some stronger evidence because they studied some 8,000 subjects of genetic pairs and the level of life satisfaction correlated with the activity levels. Want to be happier? Start walking.

Religion has a role in making people happier. Religiosity has a protective effect in warding off depression by increasing resilience. Religion seems a buffer against difficulties severe enough to restrict happiness.

A further description is in my book *Live Better While You Age*. Cheers!

Let's Awaken to Stinkin Thinkin About Wellbeing

I want to propose some corrections about thinking that I believe are germane to the nth degree. It is clear that how we reason about problems largely determines how we organize solutions to solve them. So, I reiterate: the precise process of your pondering is vital.

First, I agree that convenience is important in many parts of our lives such as shopping for many personal and household items. But our body's upkeep should be totally exempt from this mindset! Our bodies are our most important possessions, by far. Obtaining the most appropriate, best care for your body, regardless of convenience is correct thinking.

The best docs are often most inconvenient; they may not be located close. I spent time in some of the top medical centers (Mayo Clinic, Ochsner Clinic, and the Texas Medical Center) and observed that many of their patients came from distant areas, including foreign countries. I rode in elevators with movie stars and knew when some nobility or ex-presidents were in the medical clinics.

If I need a procedure that isn't minor, I go where docs are prominent. If I error, whether now or when I was in practice, I want my error to be on the **overly cautious side**. It is one of the best insurance policies one can have. Convenience and cost, **get lost**.

Many medical treatment's outcomes are greatly influenced by the rapidity with which treatment is begun. This is especially true in rapid onset conditions where the symptoms have not been present for days or weeks but have just started. Also, it is true when the initial problem seems severe, such as harsh pain, weakness, paralysis, or confusion. What?

Permanent damage can result from certain conditions in a short time and almost all treatments are to amend the damaging cause, not to restore completely damaged tissues. So, stopping the damage sooner rather than later is essential. This is especially true in our really essential for life organs such as the brain and heart. Sudden chest pain, especially in the front left area. That is likely heart pain. **Don't be a dummy!**

Correct diagnosis is essential to insure that proper treatment is begun but with the many sophisticated accurate diagnostic tools available that is less of a modern problem each passing year. Yet, if the treatment involves a major procedure, it's a different story.

Major procedures require multiple skill sets from multiple specialist physicians and you want them to be superbly skilled. I once counted the number of separate steps in a quadruple bypass heart operation; there were 1,022 steps that must be done correctly and in the proper order.

Thus, the numbers of a specific procedure done by a doctor counts a great deal. Different results are seen scientifically according to the number of a particular procedure a doctor does and that a given institution does. Go to the busiest place and the busiest doctor.

Success in Keeping One's Car Dingless: Dodging Ding Damage

You may consider this topic to be farfetched as related to health but isn't one's emotional health besmirched when a new ding is found on **your** car. It is very preventable. At the risk of seeming fastidious, the following are common sense measures to dodge ding damage.

Since different actions in our material world produce different outcomes, understanding the process is the first step in opting for a high-quality outcome. Damage to one's car from another vehicle is almost never intentional because it can damage the responsible car as well. Thus, **careless damage** is from a lack of attention, usually because of distractions.

Therefore, since we, our self-valets, have no control over the other driver's attention; we must keep a distance from the neighboring car's doors such that when fully open they will not reach our vehicle. **Got it?**

Coupes and convertibles have about 6-inch wider doors than sedans and pickup trucks even more, so allow a little more distance. I try to park next to expensive well-groomed vehicles, thinking their owners are likely to be more careful with their **"darlins"**. Damage can be predisposed by parking between two bulky vehicles in older lots that were constructed to house regular sized cars.

When I park, I avoid being sandwiched between two behemoths; I just drive on and keep searching.

Cars with children's car seats may indicate the increased chance of a ding. The door to place the child in the seat must be opened fully to properly secure the child and the parent may be distracted while doing so.

Foremost, consider parking toward the far end of the parking lot where one can get next to empty spaces. Go to an end space where one can allow extra room away from the side with a parking spot, even if empty. **Get away from the herd.**

Even with many other empty spaces, I frequently come back to find a car next to mine, so the very end is desirable. Moreover, the additional walking is healthy and the steps add up over time. When at stores where shopping carts are used, I like to park in a space beside cart return corrals but leaving space away from the opening, preferably with the passenger side closest.

Safest parking is to parallel park when such is available. It is a little more technically demanding but there is no danger of another car pulling next to yours. **Yea!**

Remember, the driver's side has a door which must open and can dent but a passenger may or may not be on board making the passenger side safer. This is often true in parking lots next to the gym or employee parking lots.

Avoiding causing dings is ethically just as important avoiding getting them. I try to park such that other's doors to not reach my car and my doors won't reach their vehicles as well. If I return and find that another vehicle is close, I open the door slowly and "get small". **Turn about is fair.**

Let's Catch Some Affection
for Perfection of Our
Body's Protection

In my opinion, the immune system is far more complex than any other bodily system except perhaps the nervous system. Every organ has immune system components included therein but the organs and areas primarily dedicated to immunity include the bone marrow, thymus, spleen, lymph nodes, and tonsils.

The lymphatic system is part of the immune system with responsibility for managing the distribution of bodily fluids as a complex drainage system and barracks for immune cells.

The circulating soldier cells include three types of lymphocytes, neutrophils, and monocytes/macrophages. **Interesting**! When a foreign substance is discovered, the lookout immune cells sound an alarm. The combat group ingests the intruders and alerts the signal corps to sound the alarm to bring in more troops as well as the bomb (antibody) makers to get busy.

It sensitizes some cells for the future producing protection termed immunity. **Amazing!** Injecting substances similar to a germ that does not make one sick producing antibody is a vaccination. Edward Jenner injected cowpox vaccine which did that and eventually cured the dreaded smallpox in 1796. His genius started immunizations, which as a single discovery has saved more human lives than any other endeavor.

During hazardous times such as Covid-19, and in future pandemics, it savvy to get personal immune systems honed and ready to protect. This is especially important in older folks and those with chronic diseases such as diabetes. Foremost, there is ample scientific evidence that moderate regular exercise for 30 minutes often will tune up immunity.

After all, exercise causes muscle alterations that the immune system repairs; consider it training drills for the white cells. **Get going for safety's sake!**

Foods with especially high anti-inflammatory and antioxidant capacity include phytochemicals such as carotenoids and polyphenols which are in veggies and fruits. WebMD lists apples, apricots, broccoli, brussels sprouts, cabbage, carrots, cauliflower, garlic, legumes, onions, red peppers, soybeans, sweet potatoes, and tomatoes as being highest.

They also list oysters, yum, as having zinc. Zinc is a mineral which boosts the immune system. One of the best boosters is garlic. **So eat up.**

Cold-eeze OTC lozenges are a clinically proven tactic to reduce the detriment of colds and some colds are from Covid. Cold-eeze has not been tested with the novel Covid but is what should help. I pop lozenges whenever I begin to feel out of sorts or have been around people coughing.

Make your overall bodily functioning better with a healthy lifestyle which includes adequate sleep. Also, stress is not good for immunity. Reduce it by thinking positive thoughts: be gratified that you are well and realize the odds are remarkably in your favor. If you are free from Covid, you are among 99%. **Be cautious but relax**.

There are some vitamins and minerals that boost immune systems, including vitamins C and D among others. Vitamin D is important now because in one study vitamin D levels were measured in patients hospitalized for Covid and those with low levels had more serious courses. Of course, these vitamin levels must not be excessive. 1,000 IU of vitamin D is good and the recommended C dose 65 to 90 milligrams daily. **Stay healthy**.

It Is High Time We Put the Sublime Back in Mealtime

The word dieting carries some distain because it requires altering one of our most vital daily activities. It is always satisfying when a desired result can be achieved by doing something smarter rather than mindlessly following rules. Counting calories can be monotonous at best. We need to realize regarding our appetites that we have inherited the pondering of our ancient ancestors which is survival.

Prehistoric meals were opportunistic occurring only when hunters had success. Those who ate more and especially consumed fat had more reserve when game was scarce and they survived. We have survivor's genes!

In the Mayo Clinic book, *Guide to Stress-Free Living*, Dr. Sood mentions how to maintain a vigorous physique by adhering to what he calls the four S principles: **slow, small, savor, and smart**.

Slow: It means to relax your eating process. Initially, concentrate on taking more chews per fork portion not just rushing with the fewest chews necessary to allow a swallow. Allow the act of mastication to provide mealtime fulfillment instead of the stuffing of your belly. Chewing satisfies, ergo, chewing gum. Also, after swallowing, allow a few seconds to expire before the next fork portion. **There is no woe with going s-l-o-w.**

Small: It means to allow just a partial filling of your fork or spoon to serve you the next bite. It will be just as satisfying and reduce your caloric intake considerably.

Savor: It means to enjoy the tastes and texture of each bite. It is fun to relish the spices, varied flavors, the content's essences, and the mouth feel of what you are eating. Doing so provides added satisfaction in consuming what will become part of you.

Smart: It means to choose what you consume according to its nutritional value, not according to its caloric content. Avoid foods that contain a lot of salt, are high in calories, high in saturated fat, or processed. Fruits and veggies are a bonus for your body, especially dark green veggies and berries.

And my bride and I add a fifth S, skip. When we have enjoyed a large earlier meal or for other reasons are satisfied, we skip the pending meal, frequently substituting popcorn.

Adopting the four S principles will allow your brain to decide sooner that you are satiated with smaller amounts and that more enjoyment accrues **especially when you stand before a mirror**. In addition, try to eat with others so it becomes a social time as well.

An added recommendation is that three meals a day is a convention from European settlers who focused on a 9 to 5 workday. The Bible has reference to two meals a day in the morning and evening. Romans ate one meal daily and eating more was considered gluttony. **Hello, fellow gluttons**. It is hard to break what you were brought up doing but consider whether you need to eat conventionally or smartly.

At mealtime, my bride and I frequently ask each other "are you hungry"? If each of us answers no, we **thankfully skip** and **do not miss** the unnecessary meal. The fat cells ante up the calories we burn until the next mealtime and shrink. **Shrink you freeloaders!**

Let Resolutions Abound and Expound Innovative Solutions

Resolutions have a unique history because the month of January named after the Roman god Janus, who is the god of beginnings and endings. Indeed, having a unique profile of two faces: one in the back of the head to survey pasts and one in the front looking to futures. Learn from your past to shape your future and thrive.

So as the phrase "New Year's Resolution" suggests, January is a wonderful opportunity to better our lives by means of thoughtful examination of our lifestyle practices and how they can be enriched. However, I robustly propose that multiple times each year everyone consider examining if resolutions would offer a better lifestyle.

First, it is important to consider what is most important in your life. What will give you the most long-term lifespan satisfaction? Consider that question sincerely which I do each time I log in another 584 million mile trip around the sun for my birthday.

My answer is a resolute retain good health and perhaps even improve it. As previously mentioned, The word "health" derives from Old English roots meaning wholeness or in olden times the state of being uninjured. Originally, the word's root meant "being fit" for life—having health was a good omen for all of one's activities. Wellbeing is a near synonym. Health's meaning, however, currently has abridged to mean freedom from physical maladies. Incomplete!

The World Health Organization defines health as: 'A state of complete physical, mental and social wellbeing and not merely the absence of disease or infirmity.' Amen!

Ask what small but meaningful improvements can I make to my lifestyle, nothing major because going overboard with resolutions is a foremost reason for resolution failure within the first month. First, realize that gaining a healthier lifestyle will have many benefits for you, your loved ones, and friends.

You will be able to function better with value-added physical, mental, emotional, or social living especially if you are older. You don't have to just let your abilities sag in some aspect of your functioning. Get going.

Carefully plan the details of how you will accomplish reaching the goals you desire and the satisfactions you will enjoy as you do so. If you are increasing your exercise routine, outline the place you will go and the times you will be there. Eat healthier diets by planning for a more nutritious regimen by serving more fish, vegetables and fruits. Reduce fatty meats, sugar, and reduce portions. Include incremental improvements over time.

A foremost New Year's resolution is to lose weight and the obvious answer is to reduce calorie intake or get your body to burn more calories, or both. There are a number of successful plans and the safest and most reliable is to join a medical weight loss clinic.

You might desire to expand your knowledge base by enrolling in courses online. I personally am going to return to a habit of reading at least one non-fiction book a week. I did that for many years but have gotten out of that habit, but will **resolve to resume** soon in January.